Thru-Hike
the Superior Hiking Trail

A COMPREHENSIVE GUIDE

**Planning, resupplying, safety,
bears, bugs, and more**

By Annie Nelson

SECOND EDITION

Publisher
North Shore Press
A division of
Northern Wilds Media, Inc.
PO Box 26
Grand Marais, MN 55604
(218) 387-9475
www.NorthernWilds.com

ISBN 978-1-7332652-1-8

Printed in Canada

10 9 8 7 6 5 4 3

Disclaimer: The author disclaims any liability for injury or other damage caused by hiking the Superior Hiking Trail. Backpacking and thru-hiking are always risky undertakings; it is up to the users of this guide to plan hikes carefully, and hike safely. The author has exercised due diligence in reporting accurate information in this guide, including researching and fact-checking all information. She assumes no responsibility for errors, omissions, inaccuracies or inconsistencies. All information is current as of the date of publication.

Dedication

This book is dedicated to my mother,
who has no plans to spend a night in a tent ever again,
yet unfailingly supports her daughter's wild, wandering ways.

This guide is also available as a digital eBook
for Kindle on Amazon. A free Kindle app can
be downloaded to any smartphone if you don't
own a Kindle tablet.

Thank You!

Your purchase of this guide supports the SHT

10% of the author royalties from this guide will be donated to the Superior Hiking Trail Association to help support and maintain Minnesota's premier long-distance trail.

Acknowledgements

Caroline Cox, a fellow SHT hiker, so thoroughly edited this guide that I owe her at least 17 favors. If you have the good fortune to meet her on trail, give her some trail magic, eh? Caroline is an amazing outdoorswoman and writer, and I highly recommend her blog, Boreal Backpacker, where she writes beautifully about her adventures and dishes out free, gourmet backpacking recipes. (Seriously, try her Taco Salad recipe. It's the best rehydrated meal I've ever had.)

My gratitude also goes to Jen Theisen, another SHT hiker, for reading the guide and providing wonderful feedback. Jen is also a High Adventure Treks leader for the Scouts, finisher of the 52 Hikes Challenge, DIY gear-maker, and prolific outdoor writer on her blog, Wandering Pine.

Thank you to everyone at the Superior Hiking Trail Association for being so supportive of this project, especially Trail Development Director Jo Swanson who read the entire guide, and shared her extensive knowledge of the trail. All hail the Queen of the SHT Trail Geeks!

Thanks also go to Kim Fishburn and Mike Ward for allowing me to reference their trail mileage tools while researching information for this guide.

TABLE OF CONTENTS

The Superior Hiking Trail

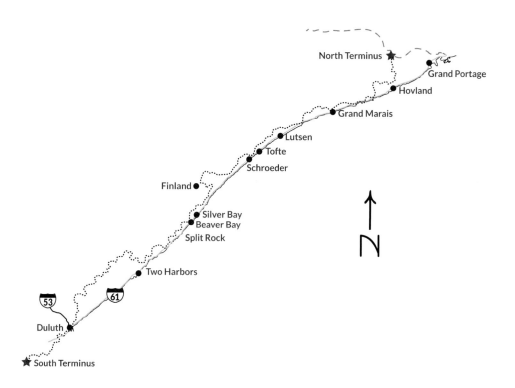

North Terminus ★

Grand Portage

Hovland

Grand Marais

Lutsen

Tofte

Schroeder

Finland ●

Silver Bay

Beaver Bay

Split Rock

N

Two Harbors

53

61

Duluth ★

★ South Terminus

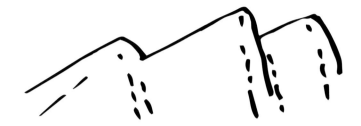

Welcome to Minnesota's premier long-distance trail

The Superior Hiking Trail is a work of art that will take your breath away with its uphill climbs and breathtaking views of Lake Superior.

The Superior Hiking Trail is a crucible in the form of a footpath that will show you the stuff of which you are made.

The Superior Hiking Trail is a love letter to the North Shore, taking you through chains of beaver ponds, bogs ringed by hemlocks and pitcher plants, groves of maples, patches of *Amanitas* mushrooms, to the peaks of the Sawtooth Mountains, and along the ancient beaches of Glacial Lake Superior.

Hiking this trail, you will learn the difference between a red and white pine, come to know what amygdaloidal and anthracite mean, and learn to sense Lake Superior's mercurial weather changes by reading the clouds.

Founded in 1986, the Superior Hiking Trail runs 297.8 miles from the Wisconsin border just southeast of Jay Cooke State Park to the Canadian border. The trail's home is the transition zone between the deciduous forests of the south and the boreal forest of the north, according to the USDA Forest Service. "Northern Minnesota is a mosaic of forest communities," the service explains on the Superior National Forest "Nature & Science" page.

Named after Lake Superior, the largest of the Great Lakes, the trail is never too far from the Grey Lady, as I call her, and she will control much of your hike. She scoffs at forecasts, brews storms in the blink of an eye, sends up walls of fog hundreds of feet tall, lies as still as glass, rages with 20-foot waves, and glitters more brightly than diamonds. She can do all of this in a single day.

The Superior Hiking Trail offers a very manageable yet exciting thru-hiking experience. Although the SHT is often called a wilderness trail and does pass through some remote areas, it offers a forgiving first thru-hike experience because you're rarely far from town and help. This trail offers both immersion in nature and easy access to resupply points, shuttles, emergency help, and replacement gear.

The trail is free to use, but far from free to maintain. Support the trail by becoming a member of the Superior Hiking Trail Association, which founded and manages the trail. A great way to earn some good karma before your thru-hike would be to volunteer on a trail maintenance project. Trail maintenance is a great work out too, so you can give back to the trail while getting in shape for your hike. Go to superiorhiking.org/join to become a member, and superiorhiking.org/volunteer to volunteer.

How to use this guide

This book is intended to be a guide for thru-hiking the SHT, not a trail guide, because a great guide, maps, databook and GPS data for the trail already exist. The Superior Hiking Trail Association released a digital, Kindle version of the Eighth Edition trail guide in spring 2019. This thru-hiking guide is meant to be a companion guide to the main SHTA guide. There is also a wonderful SHT Facebook group that has more than 15,000 members eager to share their experience with you. Much of the information in this book could also be used for planning shorter trips when you want to resupply in town.

Planning a thru-hike on the SHT can be challenging as it runs through Minnesota's famed Arrowhead region, a tourist destination. The most popular times to hike the trail — late summer and early fall — are also the height of tourism season on the North Shore. Off-trail accommodations are often fully booked months in advance, and can be quite expensive.

Part of the trail runs through the city of Duluth and does not have free campsites, which makes many hikers avoid this incredible section of trail. This guide will provide information about camping and lodging in the Duluth section in the hope that more SHT thru-hikers attempt this gorgeous section of trail.

For anyone contemplating a thru-hike of one of the many long-distance trails in America like the Appalachian Trail (AT) or the Pacific Crest Trail (PCT), thru-hiking the Superior Hiking Trail would make a great practice run to test your gear, body, and mental fortitude.

Unlike longer trails like the AT and PCT, you won't find a large cohort of hikers all setting off together in the same direction at the same time. You probably won't find a "trail family" with which to share expenses or hitch into town, but that's not to say you won't meet incredible people for short periods of time. I met a fellow female thru-hiker during my hike, Caroline Cox. We chatted for just five minutes near Carlton Peak. I was heading northbound and she was heading southbound. Since that encounter, we've reconnected online and even co-lead a group hike on the trail of members of the SHT Wild Women Facebook group.

The numerous hostels and trail-oriented businesses that exist on the AT and PCT don't exist yet for the SHT, although new hostels and businesses that cater specifically to hikers are opening every year. There are many existing outfitters and resorts that are very friendly to hikers.

This thru-hiking guide covers a variety of topics from resupplying, transportation to and on the trail, safety, weather, animal encounters, managing the bugs, and more. I hope this guide will help you stress less, and hike happier.

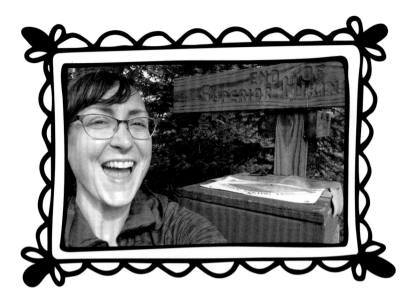

Meet the author

Hi! My name is Annie. Welcome to my book.

The first time I thru-hiked the Superior Hiking Trail in 2017, I joke that I clinched the "Slowest Known Time" record. I spent 48 days hiking the 297.8-mile trail. Thru-hiking the trail can be done much faster, which this book will discuss, but my goal was to immerse myself in the woods. I wanted to go slowly, and let my intimacy with nature develop on nature's terms.

Since 2017, I've backpacked more than 2,000 miles. In 2017, I set out on my first big outdoor adventure: a 500-mile, 75-day hike on three separate trail systems in northeastern Minnesota: the Border Route Trail (BRT), the Superior Hiking Trail (SHT), and Isle Royale National Park. I called it my "Arrowhead Amble."

In 2019, I thru-hiked the SHT a second time while hiking a third of America's longest National Scenic Trail, the North Country Trail. I made it 1,500 miles. The North Country Trail's route now includes the Superior Hiking Trail thanks to federal legislation passed in the spring of 2019.

I've hiked as many as 23 miles in a day, and as few as 4 miles during a long-distance trip. I know what it feels like to hike so far that I'm worried I've fractured bones in my feet because of how badly they hurt. I also know the joys of hiking extremely slowly down a trail, savoring each and every beautiful sight I come across.

I'm from St. Paul, Minnesota and frequently traveled to the North Shore as a kid. I learned how to build fires at Split Rock Lighthouse State Park. I grew up climbing the northwood's trees and boulders, skipping stones into Lake Superior, and trying to swim in its frigid waters before running, shrieking, back out again. At the end of week-long canoe trips to the Boundary Waters with my cousins, I never wanted to go home the final day of the trip.

I started backpacking solo in 2016 on the Superior Hiking Trail. After my fourth section hike on the trail that year, I realized I wanted to thru-hike the trail.

Thru-hiking the Superior Hiking Trail changed my life. My gratitude for that experience spawned a desire to help others successfully thru-hike the trail. I worked as a journalist for 10 years. I hope my experience as both a backpacker and a writer make this a useful, enjoyable guide for your thru-hike.

Trail Journal: The night before my big hike

I include this journal entry not as a prescription of what I think every hiker should do before a thru-hike, but rather to show how excited I was the night before my trip, what I did to prepare, and what kind of reactions I heard from people before I left.

***

7-16-17, 10 p.m.—Gunflint Outfitters Bunkhouse

Tonight is the first night of my 3-month long-distance hike through the Arrowhead region of Minnesota. My plan is to thru-hike the Border Route Trail (63 miles), then the Superior Hiking Trail (310 miles) with long hikes through several state parks added in, and then the Border Route Trail again to the Kekekabic Trail (40 miles).

The first hike of the BRT starts tomorrow with Colin, my boyfriend, thank God. The butterflies in my stomach are intense. I wouldn't be brave enough to hike this rugged trail through the Boundary Waters Canoe Area Wilderness by myself the first time.

I decided to attempt this hike back in November, and asked for a leave of absence from work in February. To my total shock, they agreed. At the time,

I was prepared to quit my job if necessary, but now I am thanking my damn lucky stars that I have a job waiting for me. I've spent at least $3,500 on the trip so far between buying new gear, taking classes, and preparing food for myself and Buddy, my dog. I've been working since I was 14 years old, that's 21 years of getting a regular paycheck. It feels terrifying not to have another paycheck coming until November. If I didn't have that job waiting for me, I'd be tempted to quit the hike right now out of financial fear.

I've been preparing for the trip in earnest since March, including buying better and lighter gear, $1,900.

I've been dehydrating food since April, thanks to a generous Christmas gift of a dehydrator and vacuum sealer from Mom.

Colin and I have been doing training hikes since March, and spent Memorial Day volunteering with a trail clearing crew on the SHT. Going to the boxing gym 2-4 times a week has me in the best shape of my adult life.

I've paid my membership dues to the Superior Hiking Trail Association (SHTA) and North Country Trail Association (BRT and Kek).

I've spent months consulting maps, guides, and online groups. I figured out where and when to resupply and listed my plan on an Excel spreadsheet. I spent the last two weeks, with tons of Colin's help, packing resupply boxes with three months of supplies. I bought the Gaia GPS app for my phone, and a satellite SOS device, the InReach Delorme SE, so I can radio for help, if needed. I even called a wilderness rescue squad to see what happens when they rescue a solo hiker off the trail who has a dog.

I consulted with Buddy's vet about his needs during the hike, things like paying attention to the condition of his feet, dehydration, and waterborne illnesses.

Colin and I took a 2-day, 16-hour wilderness first aid course that cost $240. We researched how to deal with "immersion foot syndrome," or trench foot , because the trail is so wet that some people have reported ending their hikes early due to foot issues. Lake and Cook Counties have received two inches more rainfall than average in June and July. We also went to an orienteering event to improve our compass skills, which we practiced throughout the spring.

I designed a three-month meal plan using an Excel spreadsheet, and tried to vary my foods and nutrients, and made note of when I needed to include things like tick preventative for Buddy and medications for me.

An Appalachian Trail thru-hiker named Kaitlyn even came to our house to give me a "gear edit," in which she reviewed all my gear and gave me suggestions about what to keep, what to ditch, and tips and tricks for lightening my load.

I've watched hundreds of backpacking videos, including those of a local backpacker Sean "Shug" Emery, who thru-hiked the BRT just three weeks ago. We also reviewed recent trail conditions reports on Facebook groups and the BWCA sub-Reddit.

So, we've done a lot of prep work, and I hope it's enough to make this a successful attempt of the "Minnesota Triple Crown." That's my personal nickname for hiking the SHT, BRT and Kek back to back, a play on the name for thru-hiking the Appalachian Trail, Pacific Crest Trail and Continental Divide Trail.

All of these plans and research have built in me a knowledge-base, but now that knowledge gets real-world testing.

In the months leading up to the hike, I've learned just how afraid people are of nature, of leaving behind the real and perceived safety that having four walls, a roof, and a steady job give us. These are all quotes that were said to me in the months leading up to my hike:

"Are you bringing a gun?" (Asked at least 10 times by a very concerned co-worker, who was also very excited for me.)

"If I were your father, I wouldn't let you go."

"What does your boyfriend think of this?"

"You're going alone?!"

"Are you bringing pepper spray?"

"What about bears?"

"What about ticks?"

"AREN'T YOU SCARED?"

I've been asked these questions, conservatively, at least 50 times each. People are so afraid of the woods. It is really frustrating; it feels like people are constantly trying to scare me back to my senses. But I have to acknowledge that some of their concerns are valid. An SHT hiker came down with Lyme Disease just last week. And I saw the first bear of my life tonight, the first night of the trip, here at Gunflint Lodge (in fact there were four bears in the resort tonight, a solo bear that I saw and a mother with two cubs that Colin saw down by the lake.)

Confession: I'm most afraid of straight-line winds. There were storms up here that did kill people last year. This is a dangerous undertaking, and I will be as careful as I can, but the pull of the woods is stronger than my fear. I do have moments when sheer terror unfurls in my stomach and expands until I think I'll vomit. But there are also moments when my excitement builds like a thunderstorm in my veins, guts and skin until I feel like I'll explode.

I'm profoundly grateful, happy and scared to have taken this risk.

I'm not sure when we head out tomorrow. I'm meeting with the outfitter at 7 a.m. We're getting shuttled to the eastern end of the BRT and will spend 9 days hiking back here. Colin, Buddy and I are going to wander down to the lake to see if the predicted Northern Lights are putting on the best light show on earth.

P.S. No Northern Lights tonight, but we did hear a pack of wolves howling very close by. So, yes, there are things that go howl and growl in the night.

P.P.S. According to the Gunflint staff, the howling was their sled dogs. Ha!

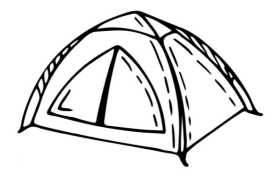

Why thru-hike?

My desire to thru-hike was born of a decade of wilderness and backpacking trips. I followed what felt like a natural progression of pushing my limits further — longer distances, solo trips, and then long-distance backpacking. My personal motivation is simple: I feel more alive and at home in the woods than I do in the comforts of modern life.

I've read the blogs and watched the vlogs of many thru-hikers who've answered this question, "Why thru-hike?" Everyone's motivation is a little bit different, but there seem to be three main categories:

- **The physical challenge:** These hikers want to test their physical limits and learn what their body is capable of doing. They are the hikers who will focus on how high they can get their mileage; how fast they can hike. They will often add physical challenges like hiking 24 hours straight, or summiting a nearby mountain even though it's not part of the main trail.

- **The mental challenge:** These hikers want to test their mental limits. They seek to learn how much mental fortitude they have when pushed past their physical limits and outside their comfort zones. They seek to test their courage and wits in the wild.

- **The spiritual sojourn:** These hikers are looking for some larger insight about their life or life as a human on earth. Some hikers knowingly embark on a spiritual journey, desiring a deeper connection with nature, or a higher power. They seek to be humbled by the trail in the best sense of the word. They are on a pilgrimage.

I think all thru-hikers experience some degree of physical, mental and spiritual growth. Thru-hikers share a desire to explore the unknown, the unknown in the natural world and the unknown in themselves.

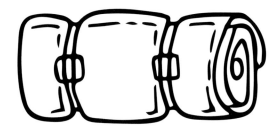

Transportation
to, from, and on the trail

Getting to your starting point on the trail can be an adventure in itself. To leave behind your vehicle and know you'll be traveling mostly by foot for an extended period of time feels exhilarating.

By plane

You can fly straight to Duluth International Airport (DLH). There are various taxi companies and hotel shuttles that depart from the airport, as well as city bus service.

It may be more expensive to fly to DLH than flying to the Minneapolis-Saint Paul International Airport (MSP) and finding a different way north.

Shuttle services and Greyhound and Jefferson Lines buses run to Duluth from the MSP airport. Groome Transport runs 15 shuttles a day between MSP and Duluth.

By train

Train service between the Twin Cities and Duluth is not available.

By bus

Both Jefferson Lines and Greyhound offer daily buses that run from various starting points in the Twin Cities to Duluth with tickets starting at $25 for a one-way ride. Both drop off at the Duluth Transportation Center at 228 W. Michigan St., right next to Canal Park, and the Superior Hiking Trail is close by. If you're not concerned about completing the entire trail, this would be a great place to start a hike as the campsites at Bagley Nature Center are only about 3.5 miles away. This would cut off the first 40 miles off of a complete thru-hike, but it sure is an easy, slick option.

To get to the southern terminus of the trail from the transit center, call a taxi or catch a ride to the Wild Valley Road trailhead. Public transportation can only get you as far south as the Fond du Lac trailhead by catching Bus 2F of the Duluth Transit authority system from the transportation center.

ARROWHEAD TRANSIT

If you catch a Jefferson Lines or Greyhound bus to Duluth, you can connect to Arrowhead Transit, which runs a weekly bus from Duluth to Grand Marais on Tuesdays and only costs $10. The Arrowhead Transit bus leaves the Duluth Transportation Center at 3:25 p.m. and arrives in Grand Marais around 6:30 p.m. This bus can pick up or drop off all along Highway 61. To drop off near or at Two Harbors, the cost is $2.50; near or at Silver Bay, $5.

To get to the northern terminus, your best option is to catch the Superior Hiking Shuttle or take Harriet Quarles Shuttle Service. Contact Harriet and the Superior Hiking Shuttle directly for prices.

Arrowhead Transit provides bus service between Grand Marais and Duluth, and back, on Tuesdays. The cost of a ticket between Duluth and Grand Marais is only $10. The bus departs Grand Marais at 8 a.m. on Tuesdays, then travels down the shore stopping at 9 a.m. in Silver Bay, 9:45 a.m. in Two Harbors, and arrives at the Duluth Transportation Center at 10:15 a.m.

The bus departs from the Duluth Transportation Center at 3:25 p.m. and arrives in Grand Marais around 6:30 p.m. The bus can pick up and drop off all along Highway 61.

For thru-hikers who would like to hike northbound to a vehicle left at the northern terminus, a good option would be to drive up Monday, arrange a shuttle pick up from the northern terminus back to Grand Marais, stay the night in town and then catch the Tuesday bus south to Duluth to start your hike. Or vice versa, thru-hikers could leave a vehicle at or near the southern terminus, ride the bus to Grand Marais, shuttle to the northern terminus and hike back to their vehicle.

Arrowhead Transit also provides local bus service and Dial-A-Ride services in communities along the North Shore. Thru-hikers could shorten the 6-mile road walk into Two Harbors by calling the Dial-A-Ride Bus to pick them up either at Press Camp Road (3.5 miles south of the Reeves Road Trailhead on Highway 2) or from Betty's Pies (2.6 miles south from the Lake County Road 301 Trailhead). Dial-A-Ride is $1.25, available 7 a.m. to 6 p.m. Monday through Friday. Arrowhead Transit requires ride requests to be made at least one hour prior to your desired pick-up time. Arrowhead Transit's reservation phone number is (800) 862-0175.

By shuttle

There are several shuttle services that cater specifically to SHT Hikers on the North Shore: the Superior Hiking Shuttle, Harriet Quarles Shuttle Service, Cadillac Cab, and Northshore Shuttles. The Superior Hiking Shuttle has a regular schedule that is updated each year. All of the shuttles are available for immediate pickups as well, or by appointment. If you run into an emergency on trail and need to get to town quickly, the shuttles will come pick you up.

Bus and shuttle contact information

Jefferson Lines: jeffersonlines.com

Greyhound: greyhound.com

Groome Transportation: groometransportation.com

Arrowhead Transit: arrowheadtransit.com

Duluth Transit Authority: duluthtransit.com

Harriet Quarles Shuttle Service: (218) 370-9164
Price varies by number of hikers and distance.

Harriet picks up from as far south as Duluth if the hiker is traveling to the northern end of the trail. She does not service Duluth to Jay Cooke State Park.

Harriet prefers reservations be done by calling or texting. She spends winters in Florida, and usually announces when she's back in town and available to shuttle on the Superior Hiking Trail Facebook group page. Harriet says, "I arrive in May with the robins, and leave in early November."

Superior Hiking Shuttle: superiorhikingshuttle.com, (218) 834-5511
Price varies by number of hikers and distance. Provides shuttle service between Castle Danger and Grand Marais May 10-Oct. 13. Shuttle service is available to the northern terminus, and non-scheduled stops by appointment.

Bob, the owner of the Superior Hiking Shuttle, is very responsive to calls, texts and reservation submissions through his website, but prefers to communicate by text as he's usually out shuttling hikers during hiking season. Contact Bob or visit the website to see the dates of operation for the shuttle.

Cadillac Cab: (218) 220-9720

Price varies by number of hikers and distance. Cadillac Cab is operated by Jeff Asmussen primarily serving SHT hikers in the Two Harbors and Silver Bay area. He is willing to shuttle the full distance of the trail for an additional fee.

Northshore Shuttles: iatonnam0972@gmail.com, (608) 921-9400

Matthew Iatonna provides shuttles in the Duluth area, and from the southern terminus all the way up to the northern terminus. For service in the Duluth area, he charges 80 cents a mile from his "point of departure," which is Superior, Wisc. For a ride to the southern terminus for a hiker in the Duluth area, the cost averages between $20-$25, he said. Matthew is also able to drop off resupply boxes to hikers, and will stop free of charge for hikers to drop off or pick up resupply boxes along the trail. For a shuttle to the northern terminus, Matthew charges $350 for up to three people, including two pets.

By automobile

DRIVING YOURSELF

If you live in Minnesota or the Midwest, hikers commonly drive themselves to the trail, and then shuttle to their starting point. Most thru-hikers go southbound (SOBO) so they can hike back to their vehicles since cell phone coverage to call for a shuttle at the northern terminus is not dependable. Many SHT thru-hikers will leave their vehicle at a southern trailhead like Wild Valley or Martin Road, and catch a ride, shuttle or bus to the northern terminus.

Leaving a vehicle at a trailhead for the length of time required to complete a thru-hike isn't without risk. There have been break-ins of vehicles left at trailheads, but very few. If you don't leave any valuables in your car while you're hiking, the risk is minimal. I met hikers who left their car midway down the trail and used it to store a resupply, which I thought was very clever.

CATCHING A RIDE

By far the easiest option is enlisting the help of a family member or friend to drive you. Check with your network to see if anyone is planning a trip near the trail around the time of your hike, or offer a family member or friend gas money and a nice reward for their help — shoveling their walk a few times during the winter, a 12-pack of beer, paying for a night in a hotel in Grand Marais.

According to Jo Swanson, trail development director for the Superior Hiking Trail Association, trailheads have been filling up with vehicles more quickly than previously. If thru-hikers can arrange to be dropped off and picked up without leaving their car in a trailhead for weeks, it would help trailhead congestion. It is still allowed to leave your car at a trailhead for a thru-hike, she said. Harriet Quarles, previously mentioned in the shuttle section, is able to store vehicles in Grand Marais for thru-hikers. Contact her for more information.

Some thru-hikers have asked other SHT Facebook group members for rides, which sometimes works, especially if you're traveling to the trail from the Twin Cities metro area. People are driving up to hike the trail every week and weekend, and are sometimes willing to help out other hikers. It never hurts to ask.

HITCHHIKING

Hitchhiking is illegal in Minnesota, which the state defines as a person standing "in a roadway for the purpose of soliciting a ride from the driver of any private vehicle." Many hikers do hitch rides without issue near the trail. I do not recommend trying to hitchhike from the Twin Cities to the trail, for example, but catching a ride from a fellow hiker at an SHT trail-head is often possible. Your decision about hitchhiking has to be personal. I opted not to hitch during my trip because I was traveling solo.

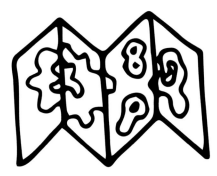

Planning your thru-hike

The details involved in planning a thru-hike can be overwhelming. I spent the final two weeks before I left with a migraine because of stress. Hindsight is 20/20; this was totally unnecessary. Before delving into the details, I want to encourage you to give yourself as much flexibility in your hiking plan as you can. The Superior Hiking Trail is so well-documented between the guide, maps, its online communities, and now this thru-hiking guide, that you can plan by section rather than by day. Find a balance between the Leave No Trace principle of "Plan and Prepare" and obsessive overplanning (like me).

Do pay close attention to the Trail Conditions page on the SHTA website, superiorhiking.org, which the SHTA updates weekly. Also read the Know Before You Go, FAQ, Thru Hiking and Leave No Trace pages on the website, which outline rules, trail safety, and more. Check the Trail Conditions page during your planning stage, right before you go, and whenever you're in town or have cell service. Take a screen grab of the web page on your phone before leaving town to reference when on the trail if you don't have service. Other hikers you meet on trail coming from where you're going will also be a good source of information on trail conditions. The woods are constantly changing: beavers flood the trail, trees come down, new reroutes are sometimes needed.

One of the best parts of thru-hiking is that you have time on your side. The luxury of free time is a rarity in our fast-paced society, and it took me a while to realize how much flexibility I really had. If you can embrace being more relaxed with your hiking plan, you will set yourself up for success.

If you're going to hike 10-12 miles a day, plan to resupply every 50 miles or so. Most hikers carry about 1.5-2 pounds of food per day per hiker, so

10 pounds of food gets a solo hiker five days of uninterrupted trail time. If you're hiking 15-20 miles a day, plan to resupply every 75-100 miles.

If you have a mileage goal for the week instead of a daily goal, you can be more flexible with yourself, the weather and any unforeseen circumstances. Most resupply options are very flexible, time-wise. Hotel reservations can be changed. Resupply packages sent "General Delivery" to post offices will be held between 10 days and a month.

To maintain the frenetic pace of our everyday lives, it's hard to avoid developing a frantic outlook on time. If you can force your mind to let go of worrying about deadlines and just focus on putting one foot in front of the other, your confidence will grow with each step in your ability to adapt quickly and successfully to changes.

Some days, you are going to wake up and discover your body is hungry to hike. You'll cover 10 miles by lunch and be amazed by how you feel ready to hike another 10. Other days, you'll wake up and be struggling by mile four, more in the mood to hang out by a babbling creek. One of the biggest gifts you can give yourself on a thru-hike is allowing your body, nature and the weather to guide your day. Sunny and feeling strong? Hike fast and far. Blisters getting excruciating? Take a rest day.

Study this guide, study the SHTA guide, sketch a general plan for your hike, but don't worry about planning your hike down to the day unless that brings you joy, or lessens your stress. You can and will figure out your hike as you go.

Trail overview

When people think "Minnesota," they don't think "mountains," but after hiking the Superior Hiking Trail, that changes.

The Superior Hiking Trail runs through the Northshore Highlands and Sawtooth Mountains, formed 1.1 billion years ago in the same geological event that created Lake Superior. Over the length of the 300-mile trail, the trail gains and loses 41,000 feet in elevation. What does that mean? You do a lot of climbing up and down on this trail. The trail is more physically taxing than many hikers anticipate.

In 2019, after publication of the first edition of this guide, the Superior Hiking Trail Association did a new GPS reading of the trail and found its true length to be 297.8 miles, not previously measured 310 miles. In many cases, other hikers and trail references will use the previous mileage of 310 miles. This guide, the SHTA's Databook and Trail Atlas (printed and digital) use the most up-to-date GPS data and other trail references will be updated in the future; the 8th Edition of the "Guide to the Superior Hiking Trail" uses the previous 310-mile measurement.

A general analysis

The Duluth section of the trail caught me by surprise: It is rugged! I had assumed this 50-mile stretch near and through the city would be easy, or involve a lot of walking on sidewalks or roads. Not so. The Superior Hiking Trail Association created a truly magical stretch of trail through the city that feels like a secret forest corridor. Houses and cars can be seen and heard, but the Duluth hiker is more often in the trees than on the street. This section offers big climbs as it runs the ridges from Jay Cooke State Park until getting north of Duluth.

The trail is its flattest between the Martin Road and the Castle Danger trailheads, about 60 miles of gentle trail that weaves through beaver ponds and young forest. The most difficult part about this stretch are the sections that follow the North Shore State Trail, a snow-mobiling trail, which can have high grass if not recently mowed.

At the Castle Danger trailhead, the terrain gets a bit more rugged as you start to get into the Northshore Highlands along Lake Superior. One of the steepest climbs on the trail, if traveling northbound, happens up to Wolf Rock just north of the trailhead.

After looping up the Split Rock river, the trail heads toward one of the most rugged sections through Tettegouche State Park. The climbs up Mount Trudee and to the Bear and Bean Lake overlooks are tough, but extremely rewarding with some of the best views on trail.

From Tettegouche State Park all the way to the northern terminus, the trail is very rugged as you climb one Sawtooth Peak after another, and climb up and down stunning river gorges. Toward the northern terminus, the trail flattens out a bit, but still offers some lung-sapping, leg-burning climbs up Hellacious Overlook and Rosebush Ridge, the highest point on the trail.

The short version? Duluth is hard. Duluth to Castle Danger is pretty easy. Castle Danger to Tettegouche is a bit harder. Tettegouche to the northern terminus is really hard.

Pros and cons of hiking northbound or southbound

Future thru-hikers frequently ask which direction is better to hike, northbound or southbound? Several things should factor into your decision.

Is one direction easier than the other? The elevation change — gain and loss — is basically the same either direction you go, according to the elevation change chart on the SHTA's website.

Is one direction safer than the other? The northern end of the SHT is the most wild and remote, meaning you are farther away from supplies, shuttles and emergency and medical help. There is less room for error during a time when you are most likely to make errors – your first days on trail – as you adjust to life on the trail.

Is there better cell service on one end or the other? Yes, the southern end of the trail has better cell service.

Is there a better time of the year to hike a certain direction? This depends on your personal skill level and tolerance of cold-weather conditions. Generally, if you are hiking in the early spring, in order to get the mildest possible weather, starting at the southern end of the trail and riding the wave of spring northward is the best direction to go. Going southbound in September and October offers the best chance of avoiding snow. If you head north from Duluth in October, your chances of getting snowed on while thru-hiking increase with each step.

Is it easier to get picked up or dropped off at the northern or southern terminus? I think people overestimate the difficulty of hiking northbound and finding a way back to their vehicle, if they aren't parked at the northern terminus. Thru-hikers understand that things will happen during their hike to alter their anticipated finish date, which is correct. They worry arranging a shuttle to pick them up before they start their thru-hike is a headache waiting to happen, or will set up a race to the finish in an effort to meet a shuttle deadline. This is also correct. And people know that cell service gets spottier the further north you get, so they may not be able to call for a shuttle once they get to the northern terminus. Also correct. But none of that means you have to hike southbound. There are several easy options for going northbound:

- Wait to arrange a shuttle pick-up from the northern terminus until you get to Grand Marais: At this point in your thru-hike, you will have completed 250 miles. You will know your hiking speed and will better be able to estimate your arrival at the northern terminus. If you plan to camp at the very last campsite on the trail, Andy Creek, you are only 1.9 miles away from the trailhead where hikers are picked up and dropped off by the shuttles. Arrange a midday or afternoon pick-up time, and you can even sleep in before climbing up to the 270 Degree Overlook, sit for an hour revelling in your accomplishment, and have plenty of time to hike back to your shuttle pick up.

- Flip-flop the last 50 miles of trail: From Grand Marais, shuttle to the northern terminus and hike back to Grand Marais to complete your thru-hike.

- Leave your vehicle at the northern terminus and shuttle and/or bus back to the southern terminus to start your hike.

Starting in Duluth offers a gentler learning curve due to constant access to supplies and lodging. Ending in Duluth means you can hike yourself right up to a great meal and easy transportation home. There is no wrong way to hike the trail. Either direction offers pros and cons, and guaranteed adventure.

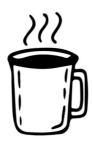

How to hike the Duluth section

As I hiked the Duluth section, seeing the Aerial Lift Bridge get closer and closer drove home the distance I was covering on my little feet. I'd never felt stronger or such confidence in my body. Before I knew it, I was walking underneath the bridge, and then it was growing smaller and smaller behind me.

If you can afford it, hike the Duluth section; it is a gorgeous, magical section of trail. Duluth does present some additional challenges because there is only one free campsite maintained by the SHTA on this 45-mile stretch, the Red River Valley campsite, which is .4 miles from the southern terminus. The next closest SHT campsite is Bald Eagle, 52.7 miles north. Thru-hiking this section requires figuring out how to manage that 52.7-mile stretch. There are five different fee campgrounds close to the trail: Jay Cooke State Park, Fond du Lac Campground (non-reservable), Indian Point Campground, Spirit Mountain, and Bagley Campground at the University of Minnesota Duluth.

If you are hiking 10 miles a day, the section of trail between Spirit Mountain and Bagley may require a hostel, motel or hotel stay as no camping options exist inside the city of Duluth. There are a couple different ways to manage this section:

Hike with your pack and pay to stay at campgrounds, motels or hotels;

Reserve a single campsite or hotel for multiple nights and shuttle to and from trailheads, bringing only a day pack (known as slack packing);

Hike 25 or 30 miles a day, and stay one night in Duluth. If you're hiking SOBO, this may be a fun way to challenge yourself at the end of your hike. You'll be in the best shape of the whole trip.

I hiked about 10 miles a day on the Duluth section and paid for five nights' accommodations. My budget for Duluth ended up being about $180. Consider making reservations in advance or arriving at non-reservable campgrounds early in the day, since accommodations fill up quickly, especially on weekends.

Below is a chart of accommodations in the Duluth area, organized from south to north. There are many hotels, motels, and AirBnbs in Duluth, but I'm only highlighting those that are close to the trail and affordable on a tight budget.

The North Shore is one of Minnesota's most popular vacation destinations. Rates for accommodations are higher during the peak demand of summer and fall, and lower during the winter. Prices are also higher for weekend versus weekday stays.

The chart lists each option's distance from the Red River Valley campsite for thru-hikers traveling northbound, and the Bald Eagle campsite for thru-hikers traveling southbound. The chart also lists how far each location is from the trail.

Duluth camping and accommodations chart

Accommodation *Nearest trailhead noted in parenthesis.*	Miles from Red River Valley Campsite	Miles from Bald Eagle Campsite	Distance from trail
Jay Cooke State Park Campground *(Jay Cooke State Park Trailhead)*	7.4	45.7	On trail
Fond du Lac Campground *(131 Ave. W. Trailhead)*	16.8	35.3	1
Spirit Mountain Campground Spur *(Loop spur)*	23.6	28.9	.6
Willard Munger Inn *(Waseca St. Trailhead)*	27.7	25	.4
Indian Point Campground *(Waseca St. Trailhead)*	27.7	25	.8
Allyndale Motel *(Cody Street crossing)*	28.7	24	On trail
Super 8 *(Haines Road Trailhead)*	32.4	20.3	1.8
Motel 6 *(N. 24th Ave. Trailhead)*	35.2	17.5	1.4
Hostel du Nord *(Duluth Lakewalk and S. Lake Ave.)*	40.2	12.5	.5
UMD Bagley Campground *(Spur to Bagley)*	43	9.7	.4

Duluth accommodation price chart*

Accommodation	Price (non-holiday)
Jay Cooke State Park Campground	$20, plus reservation fee of $10 (call center) or $7 (online)
Fond du Lac Campground	$40, non-reservable
Spirit Mountain Campground	$30
Willard Munger Inn	$74-$168
Indian Point Campground	$35-$44
Allyndale Motel	$83.93-$150
Super 8	$75-$250
Motel 6	$50-$160
Hostel du Nord	$45-$90
UMD Bagley Dorm	$25

*Tax not included.

Duluth accommodations contact information

Jay Cooke State Park Campground

780 Highway 210, Carlton, MN 55718

218-673-7000 • dnr.state.mn.us

High Landing and Ash Ridge are the closest backpacking sites to the SHT, or the main campground.

Fond du Lac Campground

13404 Highway 23, Duluth, MN 55808

218-780-2319, or 218-780-4543 • fonddulaccampground.com

Campground open early May to late October. Call for exact dates.

Spirit Mountain Campground

8551 Grand Ave., Duluth, MN 55808

218-624-8500 • spiritmt.com/campground

Campground closes in late September. Call for exact dates.

Willard Munger Inn

7408 Grand Ave., Duluth, MN 55807

218-624-4814 • mungerinn.com

Indian Point Campground

7000 Pulaski St., Duluth, MN 55807

218-628-4977 • duluthindianpointcampground.com

Campground open the week before Memorial Day until the third week in October. If reservation made, camping available May 1.

Allyndale Motel

510 N. 66th Ave. W., Duluth, MN 55807

218-628-1061 • magnusonhotels.com/hotel/allyndale-motel

Super 8

4100 W. Superior St., Duluth, MN 55807

218-628-2241 • wyndhamhotels.com

Motel 6

200 S. 27th Ave. W., Duluth, MN 55806

218-723-1123 • motel6.com

Hostel du Nord

217 W. 1st St., Duluth, MN 55802

218-940-0742 • hosteldunord.com

UMN Bagley Campground

1737 Bayview Ave., Duluth, MN 55811

218-726-6134 • www.d.umn.edu

Open year-round for SHT thru-hikers.

Suggested itineraries for hiking the Duluth section

10 MILES A DAY

Day #	Starting point	Mileage	Accomodation	Mileage
1	Southern Terminus	0	Jay Cooke State Park	9.7*
2	Jay Cooke SP	7.8	Fond du Lac	17.2
3	Fond du Lac	17.2	Spirit Mountain	24.2
4	Spirit Mountain	24.2	Super 8 Motel	32.8
5	Super 8 Motel	32.8	Bagley	43.4
5	Bagley	43.4	Bald Eagle camp	53.1

*Includes mileage for hiking from the Wild Valley Road trailhead to the southern terminus and back. Wild Valley is the closest trailhead to the southern terminus.

15 MILES A DAY

Day #	Starting point	Mileage	Accomodation	Mileage
1	Southern Terminus	0	Jay Cooke State Park	9.7*
2	Jay Cooke SP	7.8	Spirit Mountain	24.2**
3	Spirit Mountain	24.2	Hostel du Nord	40.6
4	Hostel du Nord	40.6	Bald Eagle camp	53.1

*Includes mileage for hiking from the Wild Valley Road trailhead to the southern terminus and back. Wild Valley is the closest trailhead to the southern terminus.

**Other than Fond du Lac Campground, which is about 10 miles from Jay Cooke, there really is no other option than Spirit Mountain for lodging along this stretch of the trail without getting a shuttle or ride to other accommodations in town. Total mileage between Jay Cooke and Spirit Mountain is 17.2 miles including the .6-mile spur trail up from the SHT to Spirit Mountain.

20 MILES A DAY

Day #	Starting point	Mileage	Accomodation	Mileage
1	Southern Terminus	0	Fond du Lac	19.1*
2	Fond du Lac	17.2	Super 8 Motel	32.8
3	Super 8 Motel	32.8	Bald Eagle camp	53.1

*Includes mileage for hiking from the Wild Valley Road trailhead to the southern terminus and back. Wild Valley is the closest trailhead to the southern terminus.

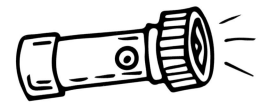

Gearing up

Gearing up for a thru-hike is a riddle, and a psychological battle. Gear is the most important safety tool hikers can have, but try to recreate too many of the comforts of home on the trail, and you'll end up with a very heavy pack.

On my first section hikes, my pack probably weighed about 50 pounds with water and food. Despite the weight, I had a great time, but I was uncomfortable while hiking. My gear was a combination of heavy hand-me-downs and gear purchased because of its cheap price.

I asked for help from the SHT's online community, even posting a picture of my overloaded pack, and it was the most humbling and fruitful pre-trip prep that I did. I was amazed to receive an offer from a recent Appalachian Trail thru-hiker to do a "gear shakedown" at my house. She went through my gear, told me what to keep, what to ditch, and even gave me recommendations on what to buy for my "Big 3:" my shelter, sleep system, and pack. Changing these "Big 3" items can make the quickest difference in the weight you carry, but they can also be very expensive. Investing in new "Big 3" gear brought their weight down from almost 14 pounds to just over 8 pounds, but cost me about $900.

I followed 75 percent of what my AT gear guru said. I still brought a camp chair that weighs more than a pound. I did not regret it for one second. My happy place on trail is in that chair while drinking a hot cup of coffee.

My best advice for gear choices is this: pick what you need versus what you want. If there is something that you still really want to bring, add it back in. Test how you handle your pack weight on short "shake-down" hikes before your thru-hike. You'll be able to lighten your load on trail by mailing gear home that you decide you don't need, or isn't worth the weight.

When deciding what you need, consider the conditions you're likely to face on the SHT. Thru-hikers should be prepared for three-season conditions even in the height of summer. The SHT is rugged. Investing in lighter gear will make you a happier hiker, help you go longer distances faster, and reduce your risk of athletic injury.

Most hikers bring a shelter, sleep system (sleeping bag or quilt and pad), pack, cook system, water treatment and storage, food storage, rain gear, clothing, footwear, trekking poles, medical kit, hygiene supplies, repair kit, technology, and navigation tools.

There are ways to lighten your load without spending a lot of money. Pare down your camp kitchen. Don't bring real books; download an eBook app on your smartphone. There is a lot of great advice online about ways to lighten your load by changing what you bring versus buying new gear. Some ultralight hikers go without items I consider basic needs like a waterproof jacket and warm layers.

Gossamer Gear, one of the companies that make super-ultralight packs, defines hikers as super-ultralight, ultralight, or lightweight based on their base weight (the weight of the pack without consumables like fuel, water and food). According to their definitions, "lightweight" means below 20 pounds, "ultralight" below 10 pounds, and "super-ultralight" as below 5 pounds. My base weight is about 18 pounds, so I can't make ultralight gear recommendations. If you are considering a weight goal, keep in mind the three-season gear you will need to stay safe on the North Shore.

Resources abound online for gear recommendations; it is an internet rabbit hole you can easily spend months falling down. If you're investing in new gear, or wanting to upgrade one or two items, I recommend starting your research by looking at recent surveys of long-distance trail hikers. The trail that offers the most similar conditions to the SHT is probably the Appalachian Trail. Thru-hikers of the Pacific Crest Trail have often already hiked the AT and are more experienced, and make more experienced gear choices. To see the top gear choices of AT thru-hikers, check out The Trek's annual survey. To see a survey of gear choices of PCT thru-hikers, check out Halfway Anywhere's annual survey. For the gear choices of some of the most experienced long-distance hikers, check out Halfway Anywhere's survey of the Continental Divide Trail thru-hikers, many of whom are finishing their Triple Crown (thru-hiking the AT, PCT and CDT).

There are many online forums and Facebook groups that discuss gear from backpackinglight.com to Facebook groups like Backpacking Gear

Reviews & FAQ and Homemade Wanderlust Backpacking Forum. A quick search of those pages will give you a lot of information.

According to The Trek's 2018 survey of Appalachian Trail thru-hikers, most hikers spent between $1,000 and $2,000 on gear. These are hikers who are planning to be on trail four-six months, compared with the average hiking time of three-four weeks on the Superior Hiking Trail. Investments in gear will last well beyond your thru-hike. If you're like me, you're going to do a lot more hiking.

There are a few tricks for saving money on gear. REI and Midwest Mountaineering have events a few times a year where they sell gently used items at great prices. Online there are several backpacking groups for buying new and used gear. My favorites on Facebook include the Backpacking Gear Flea Market, the SHT Buy/Sell/Trade/Wanted Hiking Equipment page, Twin Cities outdoors recreational equipment for sale, USA - Backpacking Gear Flea Market for Women, and Bearfoot's Hiking Gear Flea Market. Also online, you can find good deals on used gear at eBay. For new gear, there are lots of sites like Sierra Trading Post that offer deals, and massdrop.com, a website that bands buyers together to get cheaper prices. They regularly feature lightweight and ultralight gear. For Canadians, check out MEC's Online Gear Swap.

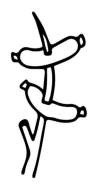

Meal planning

Thru-hikers often talk about "hiker hunger," or always feeling hungry and needing to maintain a steady "drip" of calories in order to keep their energy level up. Plan to have three meals a day with lots of snacks in between. To add calories without adding a lot of extra weight, many hikers bring packets of olive oil or coconut oil to add additional calories to their meals. Did I mention cheese yet? I brought a lot of cheese, and chocolate.

There are a lot of good websites that help with meal planning for backpacking. One of my favorites sites for creating your own dehydrated meals is the Backpacking Chef. Caroline Cox makes the best dehydrated meals I've ever had and generously shares her recipes and dehydrating instructions on her blog, Boreal Backpacker.

Backpacking grocery list

Here is a list of common backpacking foods. Deciding what food to bring depends on how much weight you want to carry. When I'm doing a shorter stretch on trail and my food bag is lighter than normal, I love bringing a couple fresh apples and carrots.

Common Backpacking Foods:

Breakfast

Instant oatmeal with dried fruit and nuts (add flax and chia seeds for extra fiber)

Bars

Pop Tarts

Instant grits w/ bacon bits

Dehydrated meal

Tortilla with cheese or peanut butter

Trail mix

Carnation Instant Breakfast

Lunch

Bars

Tortilla or flatbread with cheese and summer sausage

Tortilla with peanut butter

Tuna, chicken or salmon foil packet

Trail mix

Dried fruit

Dried veggies

Dehydrated meal

Jerky

Cheese

Dinner

Dehydrated meals

Knorr's pasta sides

Couscous mix

Mac 'n Cheese

Bean mix and instant rice

Dehydrated veggies

Dehydrated meat

TVP

Dehydrated beans

Instant mashed potatoes

Ramen

Olive oil

Coconut oil

Snacks/Drinks

Chocolate

Trail mix

Bars

Cookies

Candy bars

Gummy bears

Fruit snacks

Dried veggies

Dried fruit

Fresh fruit

Fresh veggies

Chips

Crackers

Electrolyte drink mixes

Coffee

Tea

Cocoa

Vitamins and other supplements

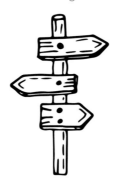

Mileage:
How far should I hike in a day?

Most SHT thru-hikers average between 10-20 miles per day. Start by dividing the total miles you plan to hike by how many days you have, but also factor in the type of hiking experience you want to have. Leisurely? Take a month. Going for a speed record? Endurance athletes frequently attempt to break the "Fastest Known Time" records for the trail and blast down the trail in a matter of days.

Many SHT thru-hikers complete the trail in about two-four weeks, depending on pace and whether they opt to do a "Traditional Thru-Hike" or a "Total Thru-Hike." A traditional thru-hike starts or ends at the Martin Road trailhead, and is about 249.5 miles. A total thru-hike starts or ends at the Minnesota/Wisconsin border and is about 298 miles, according to the SHTA.

Be honest with yourself about what kind of physical shape you're in, and keep in mind that you're likely to pick up speed as you gain fitness on the trail. If you're in good physical shape, hiking the entire trail in two-three weeks is manageable. If you've been sedentary before your hike, you may need a month.

TIP: Start your hike with lower miles for three-four days. Allow your body a "warm up" to adjust to its new job of being an endurance athlete.

Average daily mileage	# days to complete traditional thru-hike	# days to complete total thru-hike
10	25	30
15	17	20
20	13	15

When planning your hike, consider:

- How many zero or nero (nearly zero) days you plan to take.

- You will likely cover lower miles on days with significant elevation change. The SHTA's databook breaks the elevation change into 10-mile sections, which can help thru-hikers plan their hiking speed more accurately.

- Trips into towns will add to your total mileage.

- You may travel slower when your pack is heavier, for example on days you pick up a resupply.

- Accommodation can be expensive on the North Shore, and reservations at hotels and campgrounds fill up early. Sometimes it is necessary to plan mileage around accommodations booked in advance of your trip.

- What type of experience you'd like to have on the trail and your physical abilities will determine how fast you hike and how many hours you choose to hike each day. The chart below can be used to determine what average daily mileage is right for you.

Miles per hour (with breaks)	# hours hiking per day	Average daily mileage
1.5	8	12
2	8	16
2.5	8	20
3	8	24
1.5	10	15
2	10	20
2.5	10	25
3	10	30

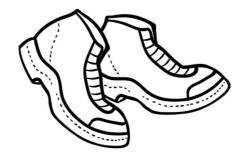

Campsite mileage
quick reference guide

The "Guide to the Superior Hiking Trail," the trail guide produced by the Superior Hiking Trail Association breaks the trail into sections. For each section, mileages are provided for the entire section, as well as distances between campsites. The guide often includes the mileage of spur trails leading off and on the section. For example, for the Kadunce River Wayside to Judge Magney State Park section, the mileage for the section includes .7 miles of access spur trail.

For thru-hikers, unless you are getting off trail to go to town, we don't usually need to know the distance of spur trails. Consequently, figuring out your daily or weekly mileage can involve a lot of math as you subtract the spur trail distances. A short cut is to use the distance between campsites. During my second thru-hike of the trail, I realized what I really wanted was a quick list of the distance between campsites so I didn't have to flip back and forth in the main guide to figure out how far apart my campsite options were, or do math with an extreme case of "hiker brain."

The Superior Hiking Trail offers 94 free campsites usually spaced just a few miles apart. There are only 16 campsites with more than 5 miles between campsites, and many of those have a state park with camping options in between them, which is why there is such a distance. The two longest stretches happen between the Hazel and Northwest Little Brule River campsites, 11.7 miles, and between the West Devil Track and North Bally Creek Pond campsites, 10.6 miles. Between Hazel and Northwest Little Brule is Judge Magney State Park, which has a fee campground. Hazel is 8.4 miles north of Judge Magney, and Northwest Little Brule River is 3.3 miles south of the park. In between West Devil Track and North Bally Creek Pond is the town of Grand Marais. The turnoff to Grand Marais on County Road 12 (the Gunflint Trail), is 3.7 miles south of the West Devil Track campsite and 7 miles north of North Bally Creek Pond campsite.

On a thru-hike, it is common to reach your planned destination for the day and realize you still have enough energy to keep hiking, if there is another campsite close by. The charts below break the trail into six sections, and list the distance between campsites for easy reference.

The charts list the distance between campsites. For example, if you are traveling northbound and want to know the distance between the Bald Eagle and White Pine campsites, the mileage placed between them is the distance between them, 1.2 miles. Quick reference guides are provided for both northbound and southbound hikers.

Northbound
Miles between campsites.

SOUTHERN TERMINUS TO TWO HARBORS

Southern Terminus → Heron Pond → Ferguson
⇕ 0.4 mi   ⇕ 4.0 mi   ⇕ 5.5 mi
Red River Valley   Sucker River   Stewart River
⇕ 52.7* mi   ⇕ 2.7 mi   ⇕ 4.0 mi
Bald Eagle   Fox Farm   Reeves Falls
⇕ 1.2 mi   ⇕ 7.3 mi   ⇕ 5.7 mi
White Pine   Big Bend   Silver Creek
⇕ 5.5 mi   ⇕ 6.1 mi
Lone Tree   McCarthy Creek
⇕ 3.7 mi   ⇕ 1.1 mi

*See "How to hike the Duluth section" chapter for more information,
including suggested itineraries, camping and lodging options.*

TWO HARBORS TO SILVER BAY

Silver Creek → Blueberry Hill → Beaver Pond
⇕ 8.4 mi   ⇕ 3.9 mi   ⇕ 1.4 mi
Crow Valley   Southwest Split Rock   Fault Line Creek
⇕ 3.2 mi   ⇕ 0.3 mi   ⇕ 4.4 mi
West Gooseberry   Northwest Split Rock   West Beaver River
⇕ 0.9 mi   ⇕ 0.2 mi   ⇕ 0.3 mi
East Gooseberry   Northeast Split Rock   East Beaver River
⇕ 0.1 mi   ⇕ 0.3 mi   ⇕ 5.3 mi
Middle Gooseberry   Southeast Split Rock   Penn Creek
⇕ 0.8 mi   ⇕ 4.6 mi
Gooseberry Multigroup   Chapins Ridge
⇕ 6.2 mi   ⇕ 1.7 mi

SILVER BAY TO CARIBOU FALLS WAYSIDE

Penn Creek

↕ 1.2 mi

Bear Lake

↕ 1.2 mi

Round Mountain
Beaver Pond

↕ 0.5 mi

West Palisade Creek

↕ 0.1 mi

East Palisade Creek

↕ 8.0 mi

West Kennedy Creek

↕ 0 mi

East Kennedy Creek

↕ 6.1 mi

Section 13

↕ 3.7 mi

Leskinen Creek

↕ 4.6 mi

South Egge Lake

↕ 0.2 mi

North Egge Lake

↕ 3.0 mi

South Sonju Lake

↕ 0.3 mi

North Sonju Lake

↕ 1.8 mi

East Branch
Baptism River

↕ 0.6 mi

Blesner Creek

↕ 2.0 mi

Aspen Knob

↕ 5.0 mi

Horseshoe Ridge

↕ 2.8 mi

West Caribou River

↕ 0.1 mi

East Caribou River

CARIBOU FALLS WAYSIDE TO LUTSEN

East Caribou River

↕ 1.4 mi

Crystal Creek

↕ 2.6 mi

Sugarloaf Pond

↕ 3.4 mi

Dyer's Creek

↕ 2.9 mi

Fredenberg Creek

↕ 1.8 mi

Falls

↕ 0.8 mi

Ledge

↕ 0.6 mi

North Cross River

↕ 0.1 mi

South Cross River

↕ 8.9 mi

Springdale Creek

↕ 2.2 mi

West Leveaux Pond

↕ 0.1 mi

East Leveaux Pond

↕ 1.2 mi

Onion River

↕ 2.0 mi

West Rollins Creek

↕ 0 mi

East Rollins Creek

↕ 4.4 mi

Mystery Mountain

↕ 2.1 mi

West Poplar River

LUTSEN TO GRAND MARAIS

A quick note about this section: There are two ways to go up the Cascade River loop. Technically, the main SHT follows the west side of the river. If you want to maintain the most pure thru-hike of the trail, follow the western side of the river. I don't think too many people would say you haven't completed a true thru-hike if you opt to use the east side, however, which has one of my favorite campsites on the entire trail – Trout Creek. I also think the eastern side has better views of the river gorge. If you want to literally go the extra mile, hike both! In this campsite chart, mileages are included for both sides.

West Poplar River

↕ 0.4 mi

East Poplar River

↕ 2.9 mi

West Lake Agnes

↕ 0.4 mi

East Lake Agnes

↕ 2.3 mi

Jonvick Creek

↕ 2.2 mi

Spruce Creek

↕ 3.2 mi

Camp Creek

West Side of Cascade River Loop

Camp Creek

↕ 3.0 mi

Big White Pine

↕ 0.5 mi

Cut Log

↕ 2.4 mi

North Cascade

East Side of Cascade River Loop

Camp Creek

↕ 3.4 mi

Trout Creek

↕ 3.4 mi

North Cascade

↕ 2.4 mi (W) or 3.4 mi (E)

North Cascade

↕ 4.0 mi

Sundling Creek

↕ 1.7 mi

South Bally Creek Pond

↕ 0.2 mi

North Bally Creek Pond

↕ 10.6 mi

West Devil Track

GRAND MARAIS TO THE NORTHERN TERMINUS

North Bally Creek Pond

↕ 10.6 mi

West Devil Track

↕ 0.1 mi

East Devil Track

↕ 2.5 mi

Woods Creek

↕ 2.4 mi

Durfee Creek

↕ 1.1 mi

Cliff Creek

↕ 2.5 mi

Kimball Creek

↕ 1.2 mi

Crow Creek

↕ 0.3 mi

West Fork of the Kadunce

↕ 0.5 mi

Kadunce River

↕ 5.2 mi

South Little Brule River

↕ 0.4 mi

North Little Brule River

↕ 0 mi

Northwest Little Brule River

↕ 11.7 mi

Hazel

↕ 2.8 mi

South Carlson Pond

↕ 2.1 mi

North Carlson Pond

↕ 3.7 mi

Woodland Caribou Pond

↕ 3.3 mi

Jackson Creek

↕ 5.1 mi

Andy Creek

↕ 2.9 mi

Northern Terminus

Southbound
Miles between campsites.

NORTHERN TERMINUS TO GRAND MARAIS

Northern Terminus

↕ 2.9 mi

Andy Creek

↕ 5.1 mi

Jackson Creek

↕ 3.3 mi

Woodland
Caribou Pond

↕ 3.7 mi

North Carlson Pond

↕ 2.1 mi

South Carlson Pond

↕ 2.8 mi

Hazel

↕ 11.7 mi

Northwest Little
Brule River

↕ 0 mi

North Little
Brule River

↕ 0.4 mi

South Little
Brule River

↕ 5.2 mi

Kadunce River

↕ 0.5 mi

West Fork of the
Kadunce River

↕ 0.3 mi

Crow Creek

↕ 1.2 mi

Kimball Creek

↕ 2.5 mi

Cliff Creek

↕ 1.1 mi

Durfee Creek

↕ 2.4 mi

Wood's Creek

↕ 2.5 mi

East Devil Track

↕ 0.1 mi

West Devil Track

↕ 10.6 mi

North Bally Creek Pond

GRAND MARAIS TO LUTSEN

A quick note about this section: There are two ways to go down the Cascade River loop. Technically, the main SHT follows the west side of the river. If you want to maintain the most pure thru-hike of the trail, follow the western side of the river. I don't think too many people would say you haven't completed a true thru-hike if you opt to use the east side, however, which has one of my favorite campsites on the entire trail – Trout Creek. I also think the eastern side has better views of the river gorge. If you want to literally go the extra mile, hike both! In this campsite chart, mileages are included for both sides.

West Devil Track

↕ 10.6 mi

North Bally Creek Pond

↕ 0.2 mi

South Bally Creek Pond

↕ 1.7 mi

Sundling Creek

↕ 4.0 mi

North Cascade River

West side of Cascade River loop

North Cascade River

↕ 2.4 mi

Cut Log

↕ 0.5 mi

Big White Pine

↕ 3.0 mi

Camp Creek

East side of Cascade River loop

North Cascade River

↕ 3.4 mi

Trout Creek

↕ 3.4 mi

Camp Creek

Camp Creek

↕ 3.2 mi

Spruce Creek

↕ 2.2 mi

Jonvick Creek

↕ 2.3 mi

East Lake Agnes

↕ 0.4 mi

West Lake Agnes

↕ 2.9 mi

East Poplar River

↕ 0.4 mi

West Poplar River

↕ 2.1 mi

Mystery Mountain

LUTSEN TO CARIBOU FALLS WAYSIDE

Mystery Mountain

↕ 4.4 mi

East Rollins Creek

↕ 0 mi

West Rollins Creek

↕ 2.0 mi

Onion River

↕ 1.1 mi

East Leveaux Pond

↕ 0.1 mi

West Leveaux Pond

↕ 2.2 mi

Springdale Creek

↕ 8.9 mi

South Cross River

↕ 0.1 mi

North Cross River

↕ 0.6 mi

Ledge

↕ 0.8 mi

Falls

↕ 1.8 mi

Fredenberg Creek

↕ 2.9 mi

Dyer's Creek

↕ 3.4 mi

Sugarloaf Pond

↕ 2.6 mi

Crystal Creek

↕ 1.4 mi

East Caribou River

↕ 0.1 mi

West Caribou River

CARIBOU FALLS WAYSIDE TO SILVER BAY

West Caribou River
↕ 2.8 mi
Horseshoe Ridge
↕ 5.0 mi
Aspen Knob
↕ 2.0 mi
Blesner Creek
↕ 0.6 mi
East Branch Baptism River
↕ 1.8 mi
North Sonju Lake
↕ 0.3 mi

South Sonju Lake
↕ 3.0 mi
North Egge Lake
↕ 0.2 mi
South Egge Lake
↕ 4.6 mi
Leskinen Creek
↕ 3.7 mi
Section 13
↕ 6.1 mi
East Kennedy Creek
↕ 0 mi
West Kennedy Creek
↕ 8.0 mi

East Palisade Creek
↕ 0.1 mi
West Palisade Creek
↕ 0.5 mi
Round Mountain Beaver Pond
↕ 1.2 mi
Bear Lake
↕ 1.2 mi
Penn Creek
↕ 5.3 mi
South Beaver River

SILVER BAY TO TWO HARBORS

East Beaver River
↕ 0.3 mi
West Beaver River
↕ 4.4 mi
Fault Line Creek
↕ 1.4 mi
Beaver Pond
↕ 1.7 mi
Chapins Ridge
↕ 4.6 mi
Southeast Split Rock
↕ 0.3 mi

Northeast Split Rock
↕ 0.2 mi
Northwest Split Rock
↕ 0.3 mi
Southwest Split Rock
↕ 3.9 mi
Blueberry Hill
↕ 6.2 mi
Gooseberry Multigroup
↕ 0.8 mi
Middle Gooseberry
↕ 0.1 mi

East Gooseberry
↕ 0.9 mi
West Gooseberry
↕ 3.2 mi
Crow Valley
↕ 8.4 mi
Silver Creek
↕ 5.7 mi
Reeves Falls

TWO HARBORS TO SOUTHERN TERMINUS

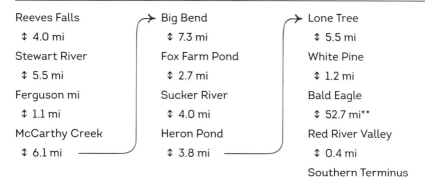

Reeves Falls	Big Bend	Lone Tree
↕ 4.0 mi	↕ 7.3 mi	↕ 5.5 mi
Stewart River	Fox Farm Pond	White Pine
↕ 5.5 mi	↕ 2.7 mi	↕ 1.2 mi
Ferguson mi	Sucker River	Bald Eagle
↕ 1.1 mi	↕ 4.0 mi	↕ 52.7 mi**
McCarthy Creek	Heron Pond	Red River Valley
↕ 6.1 mi	↕ 3.8 mi	↕ 0.4 mi
		Southern Terminus

**See "How to hike the Duluth section" chapter for more information, including suggested itineraries, camping and lodging options

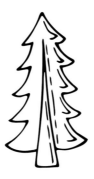

Rest days

When I arrived in Grand Marais after a week out on trail, I went straight to the Java Moose for a cup of coffee, to World's Best Donuts for a chocolate knot, and then to the Angry Trout for fish and chips and a homemade root beer. I apologize to everyone I forced to smell my hiker stink, but eating my way through Grand Marais was pure bliss. Only after I was full to bursting did I go and set up camp at the Grand Marais Municipal Campground, take a shower, and head to the laundromat. Thru-hiker priorities!

Thru-hiking is an endurance sport. You will be pushing your body in completely new ways. Walking 10-20 miles per day, you'll burn between 2,500 and 4,000 calories. You will be repetitively stressing muscles that may be more conditioned for sitting at a desk than scrambling over boulders. Your body will need rest. Your mind will need rest. Unless you are an endurance athlete or trying to complete the trail as quickly as you can, I recommend taking a rest day once every five-seven days.

You can take rest days on trail or in town. Many hikers pair their rest days with resupply days in town. The amount of time people spend in town depends on their budget and body. If you're exhausted and your feet are in constant pain, taking a full rest day can make a world of difference.

When going into town, hikers usually do one of three things:

1. Hike to town, get accomodations for two nights, and take a full rest day;

2. Hike to town, get accomodations for one night, and take a partial rest day; or

3. Hike into town, resupply, and hike back to the trail the same day.

You'll be surprised how quickly the hustle and bustle of towns will begin to feel foreign after spending so much time alone in the forest. You might find, after getting your chores done, you're suddenly ansty to get back to the trail.

Going into town to resupply can reveal some of the most interesting ways thru-hiking changes you. The level of gratitude you will feel for a toilet or hot shower will make you laugh. You will understand why sidewalks exist in a whole new way. The generosity of people excited by your adventure will amaze you.

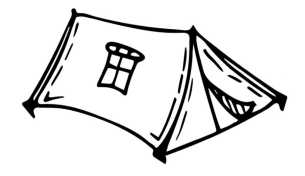

Accomodations

All of the 94 campsites on the Superior Hiking Trail are free, but the trail runs through one of Minnesota's most popular tourist destinations—the North Shore. The resorts, hotels and motels along the North Shore can be expensive, ranging in price from $60 to $250 a night.

The SHT regularly runs through state parks where you can camp, but are so popular in Minnesota that campgrounds can be fully booked months in advance. They are now 100 percent reservable, meaning you can't just wander in to a first-come, first-serve site anymore. When I was near Tettegouche State Park during my thru-hike, a ranger told me that 100 percent of the campsites on the North Shore parks were reserved that weekend.

Sometimes reserving a campsite or hotel room will be necessary, but making reservations can make you feel like you're hiking on a deadline. Hiking into town or a state park without a reservation could backfire and result in hiking a lot more miles than you'd planned to the nearest SHT site. Some hikers are comfortable leaving things up to chance, and some aren't.

State parks:
Emergency accommodation for backpackers

Minnesota's Department of Natural Resources announced in 2018 that park managers are encouraged to allow Superior Hiking Trail backpackers who are experiencing an emergency to camp for one night when campgrounds are full, according to the Star Tribune. Amy Barrett, the DNR parks and trails information officer, defined an emergency as: "a situation where personal exhaustion, injury, or equipment breakdown prevent further travel or when alternate accommodations cannot be readily obtained." Backpackers still pay the standard campsite rate.

Crowded campsites:

In 2020, the trail saw a big increase in usage. Trail Development Director Jo Swanson said future editions of the trail guide will encourage backpackers not to rely on the extremely popular campsites Bear Lake and East Lake Agnes. They will also alert people that Hazel campsite is in high demand due to it being a convenient distance for southbound thru-hikers at 19.9 miles from the northern terminus, and 11.7 miles until the next free SHTA campsites, North and South Little Brule River. Swanson says thru-hikers who can camp elsewhere should plan to do so. An option between Hazel and the Little Brule River sites is to reserve a fee campsite at Judge Magney State Park.

TIPS: The official policy of the SHTA is that backpackers must share campsites. It is not first-come, first-claim. If you arrive at a full campsite and feel you can't make it to the next site due to fatigue or safety concerns, try to make camp as close as you can to the existing pads and try to avoid damaging plants as much as possible. Jo Swanson with the SHTA said if all the tent pads are taken, as long as you set up your tent where it's possible to see the fire ring, you're good.

If it's just too crowded for you and the next site is a couple miles down the trail, keep hiking. This is another part of thru-hiking we have to accept, and grow to love. You will have days when all you want to do is stop hiking and you can't. Let these difficult moments show you that physical limits are often mental limits; nothing will make you feel like more of a badass than realizing you are stronger and more resilient than you knew.

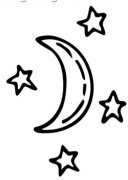

Navigating the trail: Guidebook, maps, and GPS

I was hiking through Tettegouche State Park when the trail dead-ended at a lake. The problem? I wasn't supposed to be at a lake. I pulled up the Gaia GPS app on my phone and discovered I was standing on the shore of Lake Nipisiquit. I was a half mile off of the SHT. I decided my unplanned detour was a good excuse to have some beautiful scenery with lunch.

The Superior Hiking Trail is so well-maintained, and so well-marked, that the most difficult time I had navigating was at intersections with other trails because I wasn't paying close enough attention to trail signs or my maps. Navigating the Superior Hiking Trail is not difficult.

The SHTA produces the "Trail Atlas of the Superior Hiking Trail," 41 color topographic maps of the entire trail for $24.99. A digital version of the Trail Atlas is also available through the Avenza app and are georeferenced, meaning they act like many of the available GPS apps on the market by tracking your location on the maps. The digital package of maps is also $24.99.

The SHTA also produces the "Guide to the Superior Hiking Trail," which provides descriptions of trail segments to help you know what to expect, notable features, campsites, water sources, and much more, $15.95. The latest edition is available in print and as a digital eBook. The SHTA also released a new trail reference, the "Superior Hiking Trail Databook," $11.95. Databooks are a popular reference option on other trails around America. They offer a condensed version of the "data" in a traditional trail guide. There are many stand-out features in the databook. I'm a big fan of the campsite and trailhead distance indexes, as well as the elevation profiles that are broken into 10-mile sections, which makes them much easier to understand than the trail-long elevation change map on the SHTA's website. The databook is only available in print currently, but only weighs 3 ounces and measures 5-by-7 inches, so it's easy to carry and pack.

For thru-hikers who are comfortable with digital reference materials, to keep your pack weight down, I recommend purchasing the digital version of the main trail guide, the databook, and both the Trail Atlas and the Avenza maps. If your technology fails on trail, say if you drop your phone over the edge of an overlook while you're taking that perfect shot of Split Rock River, having those physical maps and databook will make continuing on without a smartphone possible.

For hikers interested in getting Shapefiles or GPS files that can be loaded into their own navigation tools, the SHTA will be launching a data request form on its website in the future. For now, you can email info@superiorhiking.org to find out more.

I used the Gaia GPS app on my smartphone. Several GPS apps for cell phones exist. I found Gaia to be very accurate except for when the SHT shared trails inside state parks. For some reason, my Gaia maps just had blank gaps where state parks were. I was still able to use Gaia to help me figure out where I was in relation to area landmarks like lakes and roads.

Basic compass and map-reading skills are important for anyone spending time in the outdoors. There are many good resources for learning how to use a compass, from videos on YouTube to classes organized through local clubs and outdoors stores. The Minnesota Orienteering Club has resources on their website and regularly hosts educational sessions with friendly, knowledgeable volunteers who will help you learn.

Although hikers rarely need compasses on the SHT, bringing a compass and knowing how to use it is essential. Smartphones break; batteries die.

TIP: I learned during my hike that mileage counts from the guidebook often do not match the mileage counts on trailhead signs along the trail. This is due to the trail changing over the years. The SHTA plans to start updating trailhead signs soon. If you notice a discrepancy, trust the guide over the trail sign.

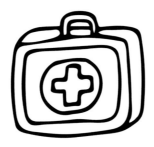

Safety on the SHT

Before my thru-hike, my imagination and fear teamed up and gave me some weird ideas. "Do bears get rabies?" I Googled. Turns out, they can. Cue mental image of a rabid bear chasing me down the trail, even though the chances of getting hit by a plane while riding a unicycle are probably greater.

Many hikers fear the animals who call the woods home, but if you look at the data, wildlife poses little risk. To increase the chances of staying safe during a thru-hike, it's crucial to distinguish between actual risks versus primal fears.

"I've never seen anyone mauled by a bear or eaten by a wolf. I'm not saying it can't happen, there are bear attacks that do occur, but generally in most cases those may be provoked by the people who get attacked," said Two Harbors Station Captain Bob Norlen of the Lake County Sheriff's Volunteer Rescue Squad. Norlen had been a member of the squad for 42 years at the time of our interview.

According to a Washington Post review of National Park Service data, the leading cause of death in National Parks between 2003 and 2007 was drowning, followed by vehicle accidents and then falls. Death by wildlife is at the very end of the list, after avalanches, pre-existing medical conditions, and heat and cold exposure.

The best source of data I've found on the leading injuries and illness among backpackers is a 2015 report by the Wilderness Medicine Institute of NOLS, which has maintained a database since 1965.

"In the context of general outdoor recreation, hikers, trekking, [...] serious trauma is rare. Sprains, strains and minor soft tissue wounds are common. Serious illness is rare," writes Tod Schimelpfenig, NOLS curriculum director, in the report. "One survey of 280 backpackers generated a medical complaint list of foot blisters, diarrhea, skin irritations and acute joint pain."

Based on this NOLS study, National Park data, and interviews with Search and Rescue teams in Minnesota, the most common injuries on trail are blisters, cuts, abrasions, diarrhea, and overuse injuries like sore knees and foot issues. Drowning and falling are the leading causes of death. "Bears kill less than one person a year in the U.S. [...] Snakes bite an average of 5,000 people a year in the U.S. Very few of these snakebites are in the wilderness and very few of the victims die," according to the NOLS report.

The key to staying safe during a thru-hike is preparation — physical and mental — and having the correct equipment, Norlen said. "Whether it's the Superior Hiking Trail, or walking around the trails at Gooseberry or Split Rock State Parks, people don't realize how rugged those trails are.

"Slips, trips and falls are the biggest things that will stop a hiker," Norlen said. "They twist an ankle, break an ankle, break a leg, fall and break an arm."

If you haven't listened to "Outside" magazine's podcast series "Science of Survival," I highly recommend it. The series makes an important point: making one mistake in the wilderness won't kill you; making several mistakes in a row kills you. I take solace from that point because if I can recognize that I've made mistakes, that I'm in danger, I may be able to rescue myself before needing to be rescued.

On Aug. 5, 2017, about three weeks into my 75-day hike, I woke to a pouring, cold rain. The temperature was in the low 50s. I realized quickly I had gear issues. My five-year-old rain shell was no longer waterproof; I hadn't tested it before I left. My only warm layer was a down coat, which I didn't think would keep me warm when wet, so I didn't wear it.

My hands were freezing. Cold water was running down my body; I was soaked head to toe. I remember taking a break beneath a spruce tree and noticing how badly I was shaking. The wind was fierce, whipping away my body heat. I realized slowly that I might be in danger of developing hypothermia. "But it's August!" I thought.

I learned later that a local YouTube vlogger named Rory Anderson (Bigfoot) was attempting an FKT of the SHT that week. He ended his attempt early the same day I was huddled under that spruce because he believed himself to be at risk of hypothermia.

Mistake one? Not testing my rain shell before my hike. Mistake two? Not having a warm layer that could get wet. I was on the verge of making my biggest mistake: I was ignoring the signals my body was giving me because I thought hypothermia couldn't happen in August.

I pretty much ran the last couple miles to camp. After setting up my tent, I dove inside my down quilt. I took more than an hour to warm back up. At my first opportunity in a town, I added a fleece sweatshirt back into my kit, which will stay warm when wet, and purchased a new rain shell.

"Time is of the essence in those situations," Norlen said. "It doesn't take long if you're cold, wet and the wind is blowing to get into hypothermia."

Let's review some of the biggest dangers on the SHT, and safety recommendations from Search and Rescue squads in the area, the National Weather Service, and others.

Major dangers on the SHT

Each trail has different hazards. On the North Shore, hikers don't have to worry about poisonous snakes or desert conditions, but they do have to deal with dangerous weather, dramatic temperature changes, insects that carry diseases, and more.

Please don't let this list scare you out of thru-hiking. The chances are very low that you will be confronted with any of these dangers, and the best way to manage them is to educate yourself about how to deal with them.

FALLING

The Superior Hiking Trail runs through the ancient Sawtooth Mountains. The trail is beautiful, muddy, rugged, and crowned with regular breathtaking views of Lake Superior from the tops of huge cliffs. What is it about a 500-foot drop off that mesmerizingly pulls you to the edge to look over? When I hike alone, I try not to get within 10 feet of the edge. I'm being super cautious, but rock isn't as stable as it looks, and Lord knows neither are my feet.

In June 2018, Pat Ditlevson, a regular visitor and hiker on the North Shore, fell into the Cascade River near the SHT and went over two waterfalls before catching herself on a rock. Ditlevson had hiked these trails many times. "I was on a rock ledge looking over the falls, [...] and my knee gave way when I stepped on some loose rock and I fell into the river, just before the two big falls," Ditlevson said in an interview with WTIP. She added that an EMT responder told her she was the only person to go over the falls and survive, to that responder's knowledge.

You will hike this section of trail and many other stretches along rivers. Take nine minutes and listen to WTIP's interview with Ditlevson about her harrowing ordeal.

Cliffs don't present the only falling danger. Recently, Tettegouche State Park installed a set of stairs on a legendary part of the trail, the "Drainpipe." The decision was controversial amongst hikers who want the ruggedness of the trail protected. I almost fell down the Drainpipe on my thru-hike, so I understand why the park made that call. The Drainpipe was incredibly steep and covered in pea-sized gravel, like trying to walk downhill on marbles.

GETTING LOST

Although the trail is well-marked, one of the most common causes of rescue on the North Shore is a lost person, said Norlen and two other deputies who coordinate search and rescue operations in Cook County, Chief Deputy Will Sandstrom and Deputy Chris Schrupp. For tips on navigating the trail, read the Navigation section.

The best way to prevent yourself from getting lost is to stay on the path, Sandstrom said. "Once you feel that you're lost, stay put. Don't keep moving, because in most cases, you're going to get more lost," Norlen said. "If you're carrying your GPS and you have route plotted, follow your GPS, but always have a compass in addition to your GPS, just to verify your position: north, south, east, west."

In 2013, on the Appalachian Trail, Gerry Largay stepped off the trail to go to the bathroom, got turned around, and got lost in dense forest. She tried to text for help, but had no cell service. She survived for 19 days, according to her journal. Search and Rescue searched for Gerry for a full week; her body was found two years later. The AT is a very busy trail, just like the SHT, and Gerry had already hiked 900 miles before getting lost. Losing the trail can happen even to experienced hikers.

If you get lost, follow the U.S. Forest Service's STOP plan: Stop, Think, Observe, Plan. Stop and stay calm; panicking can scare us into making bad decisions. Think about how you got to where you are. Are there landmarks nearby you can use to navigate back to the trail? "Don't move until you have a specific reason to take a step," the forest service says. Observe: Use your compass to determine which direction you're facing. Can you take a bearing using nearby landmarks? If hiking with GPS, drop a waypoint as soon as you figure out you're lost. Consult your maps and GPS and see if you can navigate safely back to the trail. Finally, plan: If you're confident of a route back to the trail or a road, try to self-rescue. If you're unsure, injured or near exhaustion, stay put. Try to find a clearing nearby in which to set up camp, and put bright clothing or other items you don't need to stay dry and warm around your tent so you will be more visible to rescuers.

The two most important safety techniques are staying on the trail and telling someone your hiking plan, Sandstrom said. The most common search and rescue calls are related to lost hikers or overdue hikers, Schrupp said.

"Someone goes off trail and they end up getting hurt, twisting a knee," Sandstrom said. "Stay on the designated paths and trails. Leave a copy of your itinerary with someone else. Let them know if you're going to do 3 miles a day, 5 miles a day, how many miles you're going to do a day. Then we have a starting point instead of looking for a needle in a haystack."

Ask someone at home to be your backup, someone who will call 911 if they haven't heard from you by a designated time. Let your backup know the name of the trail, which direction you'll be hiking, how many miles you expect to hike each day, and when they should expect to hear from you. For example, if you've just resupplied in Silver Bay and plan to resupply again in Grand Marais in six days, let your backup know if they haven't heard from you by the afternoon of the seventh day that they should call 911.

How much extra time you give yourself to make your destination before triggering a rescue call is a personal decision that must be based on what kind of risk you are willing to take. If you break your leg, you'll survive for a couple days without rescue. If you fall and gore yourself in the abdomen with a branch, you likely won't survive without immediate help.

Unless you somehow get separated from your pack or are fatally injured, you should have everything you need to keep yourself alive for a number of days if you get seriously injured or lost. The chances of other hikers being able to assist you are very high on the SHT because it is such a popular trail.

Technology is making us safer in the backcountry. I recommend investing in a satellite SOS device like an InReach Delorme, which allows you to signal for help, and text specific information to rescuers. This tool is especially powerful for solo hikers.

DROWNING

The leading cause of death in the wilderness is drowning, according to NOLS. There are many opportunities to swim along the trail, from the frigid waters of Lake Superior to the Caribou River.

There are a lot of signs in the state parks on the North Shore that warn about drowning risks along the rivers. At Temperance River State Park, signs warn people not to swim where the Temperance River and Lake Superior meet due to strong, unseen and unpredictable currents. Heavy rains can also create suddenly dangerous conditions. People die each year on the North Shore by getting swept downstream.

There are currently three unbridged water crossings on the trail — the Encampment River, the Split Rock River, and Trout Creek. All are avoidable by following SHTA reroutes. The SHTA constantly reassesses the trail's needs, said Trail Development Coordinator Jo Swanson. After the bridge over the Encampment River was washed out for the fourth time, Swanson said the SHTA accepted that Mother Nature won that round. "At least 95 percent of the time, the Encampment is easy to cross and the worst that would happen is you may get your feet wet. But during spring snowmelt season, or after a heavy rainstorm, fording any waterway is generally too dangerous," Swanson said.

Swanson advises hikers to be aware of their ability level with water crossings, and make common-sense decisions about when to do a crossing. On my thru-hike, I forded all three of the river crossings. The Encampment River and Trout Creek crossings were easily made, and my feet stayed relatively dry thanks to stepping stones. The Split Rock River crossing was scarier. We'd had rain for the previous two days. As I hiked up the west side of the loop past roaring waterfall after roaring waterfall, I was really questioning my decision to try and ford a fast-moving river the first time, and solo. There is a campsite just before the crossing and I decided when I got there, if conditions looked unsafe, I'd camp there for the night and hike back the next morning. I was not going to risk doing a dangerous river crossing alone. When I got to the crossing, there was a group of hikers on the other side that included a former SHT thru-hiker. When he saw how nervous I was about getting across the river, he offered to help and came out to meet me halfway. I got across just fine, but there were several deep holes and unseeable crevasses perfect for getting a foot trapped.

The best advice I've found about water crossings is this: Unclip all your pack straps — hip belt and chest strap — so, if you do fall in the water, you can get out of your pack so it doesn't drag you underwater. Go very slowly so your foot doesn't get trapped in between rocks on the river bed. If your foot is trapped and you get off-balance, the force of rushing water can push you off-balance into the water, and pin you there. If you fall, flip onto your back with your feet facing downstream, which reduces your risk of hitting your head on a boulder. If using your trekking pole for stability, point it downstream so the force of the water doesn't push the pole upward suddenly and throw you off balance.

As far as knowing when it's safe to cross, I follow this rule: If the water is deeper than your knee, it is only safe to cross if its moving more slowly than you can walk. The trouble with this rule is most river water is not clear; you can't see the bottom. The water could be 6 inches deep, it could be 6 feet deep. Due to the nature of river erosion, there can be deep channels that open up suddenly beneath you, and deep holes where the water is caught in a bend. If the water is moving faster than you can walk and you can't see the bottom all the way across to know its depth, don't risk it. None of the suggested reroutes by the SHTA are longer than a couple miles. Risking your life to save a couple miles is definitely not worth it. After speaking with the SAR teams for this guide, I have new respect for, and fear of, the North Shore's stunning river gorges.

INJURIES

When hikers go too hard too fast, they go home early. The SHT trail sets hikers up for a unique type of failure when it comes to athletic injuries and blisters. The trail is only 300 miles long, which many people can hike in just a couple weeks, but to do so requires hiking about 20 miles a day over ankle- and knee-twisting terrain. Unlike longer thru-hikes when people have three-seven months, there is no "warm up" period on the trail. SHT thru-hikers usually don't have time to take several rest days when injured like 25 percent of AT thru-hikers do.

When I was camped out at the Stewart River site, a young woman came into camp to ask me how far the next campsite was. She was pacing back and forth. "Today's my first day on trail and I've already hiked 20 miles," she said. "My legs are cramping up, so I can't stop moving."

She continued on. If she'd been charged by a moose further up the trail, how would her cramping legs have impacted that situation? How would stiff legs and sore muscles affect her ability to maintain her balance while hiking over boulders and tree roots the next day?

"Don't get yourself into a position where you're not going to be able to continue hiking," Sandstrom said.

To avoid athletic injuries, assess your fitness level honestly. If you're not in the best shape, completing a thru-hike in two weeks is not very likely. If you've only got two weeks to hike and you doubt you can do the whole trail, that's OK. Take the two weeks and start with 8-10 miles a day for a couple days, and then decide if your body feels up to hiking longer distances. If you can't thru-hike, just see how far you can get. The distance you hike is only one part of the experience.

WIND STORMS

After seeing the level of destruction caused by 2016 storms in the BWCA, my No. 1 fear in the woods is being caught in a straight-line wind storm. On the Border Route Trail, I hiked past Duncan Lake where Craig Walz died during the wind storms of 2016. The forest around the lake looked like a bomb had gone off. "We have responded to big wind storms when trees have fallen on tents, and people did not survive," Sandstrom said.

"In 1999, we had a huge straight-line wind storm in the BWCA, and a lot of people had to be rescued; we had a lot of injuries from people being in tents underneath trees," Norlen said. "In those situations, you have to get the tents out from underneath the trees and get into the biggest open area that you can."

If you can't find an open area nearby, Norlen and Sandstrom both recommended getting into a ditch or depression in the ground so that falling trees are less likely to hit you. Another option is to get into stand of younger, smaller trees that are less likely to hurt you if they fall, and may even catch or slow down bigger trees, giving you more time to get out of the way.

My plan will be to move my tent to the most open area I can find, but also to stay outside of the tent to spot falling trees. Even if it's pouring rain, I'd rather be soaked but alive. Most storms pass quickly.

Even if storms aren't in the forecast and skies are clear when you're setting up your tent, hammock or tarp, try to pick as safe a location as possible. Look up into the trees to scout for "widow makers," big, broken branches hanging in the tree, or dead branches that look likely to fall if a big wind came up.

THUNDERSTORMS

The National Weather Service does not mince words when describing the danger of thunderstorms: "No place outside is safe when a thunderstorm is in the area," according to the NWS's Lightning Safety brochure. "Go indoors!" Well, when you're 15 miles from the nearest town, going inside isn't an option.

Being struck by lightning is incredibly rare on the North Shore, said Norlen, Sandstrom and Schrupp. Schrupp said in his six years coordinating search and rescue operations, he's never gotten a lightning strike call. Norlen said a few years back, he was aware of a lightning strike incident that did not end well, but he said your chances of being struck by lightning are about equal to winning the lottery.

According to the NWS website, there are actually five different ways to be struck by lightning: direct strike, side flash, ground current, conduction, and streamers. In other words, lightning doesn't just come from above, it can also come from below, the side, and jump from trees and metal objects to strike you.

The NWS estimates 300 people are struck by lightning each year, and only 30 die. When you consider that millions upon millions of people get caught in thunderstorms each year, the probability of getting struck by lightning is vanishingly small. Even so, there are some things you can do to keep yourself safer in a thunderstorm. Here is what local SAR members, the National Weather Service, and the North Country Trail Association advise you do during thunderstorms:

- Avoid open areas; don't be the tallest thing in the area.
- Stay away from isolated tall structures like utility poles, cell towers, and tall trees.
- Don't pitch your tent on top of tree roots.
- Avoid metal conductors like railings and wire fences.
- If in a group of people, spread out 15 feet apart. This prevents multiple people from being struck.
- Don't lie down, and avoid touching the ground if possible. If not possible, squat with your feet and buttocks close together. Sit on your pack, unless it has metal components. In your tent, squat on your pack or sleeping pad.
- Avoid ridge tops or get down as fast as you can if a thunderstorm starts while you're hiking a ridge.
- Cell phones and hand-held radios with short rubber antennas are safe, but avoid using phones or radios with long antennae.
- If the hair on your body stands on end, this means there's a high probability of a lightning strike happening nearby and soon.
- Take shelter indoors or in vehicles when possible.

HEAT AND COLD EXPOSURE

HEAT: On my way to Ely's Peak, I ran out of water. The day was blisteringly hot for Duluth with a temperature in the high 80s. I was walking on an old rail bed converted to trail with no shade. According to my map, I would have to get over Ely's Peak and back down before there would be a creek.

By the time I got to the top of Ely's Peak, I had a bad headache and was feeling pretty gross. I recognized that the heat was starting to get to me, and I was likely dehydrated. Since water was still a mile or two down the trail, I decided to take a short break in a small patch of shade to give my body a break since I couldn't give it water. I wasn't in real danger as Ely's Peak area is a very popular day-hiking destination, and there were people everywhere; I could've asked for water.

According to the NOLS study, dehydration, hypothermia, heat illness and cold injuries don't even make the top 10 list of most common back-country illnesses, which they credit to good education. Most of us know how to spot these conditions and respond to them in the moment.

Symptoms of heat exhaustion include: weakness, fatigue, muscle cramps, heavy sweating, cold and clammy skin, fast but weak pulse, and fainting, according to the CDC. The CDC recommends seeking medical help if you are throwing up, or symptoms don't improve with rest and water after an hour. Heat stroke is a medical emergency, and medical help should be obtained right away. Symptoms of heat stroke include: a body temperature of 103 degrees or higher, hot skin, fast and strong pulse, headache, dizziness, fainting, nausea, and confusion.

COLD: Conditions on the North Shore can change rapidly due to lake-effect weather. Sunny, 75-degrees weather can change suddenly to pouring rain and gale-force winds with a 20-degree temperature drop in the blink of an eye.

The risk level of hypothermia depends on the season, the weather, and gear. During shoulder season — April-May and October-November — weather can be more dangerous. Snow can fall in May and September.

"We had a situation, about 15 years ago, we had some people who were hiking in Gooseberry State Park and they got turned around. It was cold. We looked for those people for two days. We found one gentleman and he was very hypothermic. His partner, we found him a day later, and unfortunately he was dead. He was down to his underwear, and had been running around in the woods. That's one of the things that happens, people think they're hot when they're cold and they start taking off their clothes, but those situations are very rare," Norlen said.

Hypothermia happens when your core temperature drops to 95 degrees or below, and it starts to affect your thinking, which makes the situation worse. NOLS says the best clues for diagnosing hypothermia include an "impaired ability to perform complex tasks, fine motor shivering, apathy, confused and sluggish thinking, slurred speech, and 'the umbles' (stumbling, mumbling, bumbling, fumbling, grumbling)."

UNDER- OR OVER-HYDRATING

Hydration can be tricky on trail. Most hikers know to drink a lot of fluids to prevent dehydration. Drinking more water than you're sweating out and not eating enough salty foods can lead to a condition called hyponatremia, which is equally dangerous. Hyponatremia happens when the concentration of salt in your blood is abnormally low, according to the Mayo Clinic. Symptoms include nausea, vomiting, headache, confusion, muscle weakness or cramps. Symptoms of dehydration and hyponatremia can be similar.

The best way to distinguish between the dehydration and hyponatremia is noting your level of water intake, and urine color. "Monitor your urine output for color and quantity—dark urine is a sign of dehydration, as are fatigue, irritability, poor thinking, thirst and headache," NOLS recommends. Drinking water and resting are the best treatment. If you're not thirsty, your urine is clear, and you've been drinking a lot of water, hyponatremia is the likely culprit.

As a general rule, keep your water bottle in an easy-to-reach location to encourage yourself to stay hydrated. If you find that you are drinking a lot of water and still feeling dehydrated, consume salt to keep the water in.

The fourth day of my hike, I was suddenly so weak that I couldn't hike. I had to lay down on the trail for a full hour before accepting that I couldn't go on. It was my boyfriend who figured out what was happening. I was hyponatremic — my salts and electrolytes were too low. We'd learned in a wilderness medicine class that hyponatremia often looks like dehydration. If we had misdiagnosed my symptoms as dehydration and I'd drank more water, a mild medical condition could've turned into a medical emergency. Severe hyponatremia symptoms include seizures and coma.

I'd been drinking a lot of water, and my urine was clear. How did I know it was clear? WARNING: This gets a little gross. I peed into a clear Ziplock baggie. I stopped drinking water, and started drinking small amounts of salted Gatorade. Over time this made me feel a little better, confirming that mild hyponatremia was likely the issue. We had to take a full, unplanned rest day on trail before I felt well enough to hike again.

When I'd packed for my trip, I'd made my own "healthy" meals that had a low salt content. I don't like eating very much salt in regular life, and wanted to avoid salty, pre-packaged dehydrated backpacker meals. I had no idea how necessary salt is to stay healthy while long-distance hiking. For the rest of my trip, I made sure to eat a lot of salty snacks and electrolytes.

WATER-RELATED ILLNESS

Beaver fever is a common nickname for Giardia, a gastrointestinal illness contracted from drinking unfiltered water, because water contaminated by animal waste usually causes the illness. "The risk of diarrhea was greater among those who frequently drank untreated water from streams or ponds," according to the 2015 NOLS report.

Along with parasites, unfiltered water can also contain chemicals like defoliants used in forestry and farm run-off. One of Minnesota's 24 Superfund sites is on the St. Louis River, which runs through Jay Cooke State Park, though the site is not adjacent to the SHT. None of the water sources along the SHT are considered dangerous if water is filtered.

TICK-BORNE AND MOSQUITO-BORNE ILLNESSES

Ticks in Minnesota carry a number of nasty diseases: Lyme Disease, Anaplasmosis, Ehrlichiosis, Powassan Virus, and more, according to the Minnesota Department of Health. Mosquito-borne illnesses are rare in Minnesota compared to the tropics, but mosquitoes can carry West Nile Virus, and several viruses that can cause encephalitis.

During the summer of 2017, the bugs were horrendous due to higher than average rains. I found bug repellant (even 100 percent DEET) to be almost useless in these conditions. Instead, I used a head net, wore my raincoat if the mosquitoes were especially maddening, and tucked my pants into my socks to prevent tick bites. I diligently checked myself each night for ticks. I only found five ticks on me during the 75 days I spent hiking.

According to the Lyme Disease Research Center at Johns Hopkins University, about 300,000 people in the United States contract Lyme each year, and the riskiest time to contract Lyme is late spring and early summer.

SUDDEN HEALTH CONDITIONS OR PRE-EXISTING CONDITIONS

"A lot of injuries we have are related to people not being physically prepared for that hike. [...] They haven't hiked 10 or 20 miles in their life, or they haven't done it in a long time, and end up having a heart attack on the trail," Schrupp said.

It wouldn't be a bad idea to get a check-up before attempting a thru-hike on the SHT to make sure you don't have any unknown pre-existing health conditions. If you have known health conditions that require medication, "make sure the medication is stored in a way that it won't be easily lost," Norlen said. If your medical history includes previous injuries, like ankle sprains, make sure your first aid kit is supplied to deal with the possibility of re-injury.

WILDLIFE

On a hike with my best friend in the Colorado Rockies, a ground squirrel ran straight up her leg and bit her finger to get her to drop the trail mix in her hand. We all screamed, and then started laughing. "That hurt!" she yelled; She did not appreciate that we found her animal attack hilarious. By far, the most ferocious animal I faced during my thru-hike were the chipmunks. My favorite nickname for them is "Timber Tigers."

The most painful wildlife encounter you're likely to have on the SHT, and most dangerous if you're allergic, are with hornets and wasps. They love building their nests underneath bridges on the SHT, and in summer you'll see suspected hive locations listed on the Trail Conditions page on the SHTA website. Every year, numerous SHT hikers report being stung on the Facebook group page.

Bears kill fewer than one person a year, according to data reviewed by NOLS. But reports of bears visiting campsites on the SHT has been increasing. Campsites where bears were spotted included Section 13, Bear Lake, and Lake Agnes, all very popular sites. Properly storing food and smellables is crucial.

"A bear is more afraid of you than you are of it," Schrupp said. "If you see a mom and cubs, if you provoke it, it might come after you, but I'd be more afraid of a moose. A moose will charge you, especially if it's around its calf."

The only bear I saw during my hike was at the Gunflint Lodge. An employee told me someone had left a blueberry pie to cool on a windowsill a few days earlier, the bear had eaten it, and now it was visiting the resort every night looking for another pie. If you do encounter a bear, here are some recommendations for how to handle the situation:

- If you're not being charged, don't run; running can trigger a bear's prey drive.

- Do not get between a mother bear and cubs.

- If you see a bear and it has not seen you, back away slowly while facing the bear.

- If you see a bear and the bear has seen you, make yourself look big and make noise. Make a quiet noise at first so you don't startle the bear, but to make sure it knows you are there.

- If attacked, do not play dead; that practice applies to grizzly attacks, not black bear attacks. (There are no grizzly bears, or brown bears, in Minnesota).

- If attacked, fight back and aim for the bear's eyes and face. Fight for your life.

The park rangers I spoke to during my hike were not very concerned about bears, but had a healthy respect for moose. "My advice to anyone who meets up with wildlife, back away slowly, that's about all you can do," Sandstrom said. "One of our deputies encountered a mother moose and calf on the Border Route Trail, she turned toward him, laid her ears back, and put herself between him and the calf. He backed away slowly, not panicking, not running away. He got lucky and the moose stayed where she was and didn't pursue.

"Wolves are afraid of people. Bears too. Mountain lions are in the area. Sightings are few and far between. I haven't heard of anyone encountering one on the trail. They're afraid of people, too," Sandstrom said. "If people bring their animals along, that's a different story. Wolves were attacking dogs when their owners were 5 feet away. Dogs are going to attract wolves. Wolves view dogs as a threat; they're another wolf-like animal in their territory." This is another good reason to keep dogs on a leash, which the SHTA asks hikers to do.

PLANT IRRITANTS

There are two main plant irritants on the SHT: poison ivy and wild parsnip. This book is not intended as a field guide and will only provide general information about the plants' location on the SHT and effects.

The saying "leaves of three, let them be" describes poison ivy. Fortunately, SHT hikers do not need to know how to identify this plant, since the only point on the trail where poison ivy grows—the Crow Creek crossing just east of Two Harbors—is well-signed. If you brush up against plants here, wash the contaminated area immediately in the creek to avoid a rash.

Wild parsnip "is the same common vegetable available in nearly every grocery outlet in the country," according to Samuel Thayer in The Forager's Harvest. The plant is considered invasive and, similar to many other invasive edibles, was initially brought to North America for cultivation. Wild parsnip causes a rash, similar to a burn, when sap gets on your skin and is exposed to sunlight. Thayer describes his own experience with "a painful rash or large blisters that made a case of poison ivy seem enviable."

Identified populations of wild parsnip are located on the SHT along the Cascade and Beaver Rivers and the Duluth Lake Walk, on Grand Ave across from the Spirit Mountain parking, and in Jay Cooke State Park, according to Early Detection & Distribution Mapping System (EDDMapS). Several additional populations are near the SHT, especially in Duluth. These areas are unsigned and populations are likely to spread because wild parsnip is invasive.

While knowledge of plant irritants is an asset, common sense is generally sufficient: If you avoid walking off-trail through plants you can't identify, your chances of developing a rash are low. Keen botanists and foragers may be interested in learning to identify these plants, as well as plants that can treat rashes—the most common on the SHT is jewelweed.

Who will rescue me? How much does it cost?

Search and Rescue squad members are volunteers. Sheriff's departments in Minnesota are mandated by state law to find someone lost or deceased in the woods. You will not have to pay for rescue services until an ambulance or other emergency medical transportation is needed. Search and rescue is funded through law enforcement funding.

"A lot of the calls are lost hiker, overdue hiker, or overdue canoeist from the Boundary Waters, someone who should've been out yesterday. We'll send people in, we'll try to figure out where they went in and we'll go search for them," Schrupp said. "SAR is also responsible for lost snowmobilers, people lost on a boat, and ATV. If there is a drowning, SAR also goes out and drags for the deceased bodies."

Schrupp said Cook County has 49 or 50 SAR members across the county. "(Search and rescue) is expensive. It takes a lot of manpower. All of our SAR folks are volunteers, and search and rescue operations take them off their jobs."

"We do this out of dedication and commitment to help our citizens and visitors to Lake County that are in a time of need," Norlen said. "We get a lot of satisfaction in helping, providing care, and making sure people are safe."

2018 SAR DATA FOR COOK, LAKE AND ST. LOUIS COUNTIES

In 2018, Cook County had 12 Search and Rescue (SAR) calls. Of those 12, seven calls were for a lost or overdue hiker, three were for injuries, and two were rescues, according to data provided by the Cook County Sheriff's Department. In six of the seven lost hiker calls, the hikers were found or self-rescued. Cook County Search and Rescue responded to a capsized canoe call in the BWCA and one person drowned in that incident. The drowning was the only incidence of death recorded by Cook County in its 2018 SAR data.

In Lake and St. Louis Counties, the rescue squads track their data a little differently, and respond to many situations not related to hiking like traffic crashes, boating accidents, ATV and snowmobile accidents, and more. In Lake County in 2018, the SAR responses that may have involved hikers included 85 medical-related responses, 11 search and rescue operations for lost or injured persons in wilderness areas, eight general public assistance calls, and two rope rescue operations.

In a Feb. 21, 2019 post on its Facebook page, the St. Louis Rescue Squad reported doing "73 searches, 46 rescues, five rope rescues, and one plane crash," in the woods. "On the water we responded on 10 water fatality recoveries, but made a critical difference in the live rescue of 22 others. We performed two heavy extrications, and led eight remote helicopter landing zones."

Safety gear

All of your gear is a safety device, really. Clothing insulates us from the cold, water filters prevent water-borne illnesses, and our shelters keep us out of the elements. Food is fuel, but also keeps us strong and thinking straight.

Here is a rundown of some gear specifically designed for safety purposes. I'll share my experience with gear if I've used it.

PERSONAL LOCATOR BEACONS (PLBS) AND SATELLITE COMMUNICATORS

There are a number of satellite SOS devices on the market, which allow you to signal for emergency help — medical or rescue — without having cell phone coverage. I carried a Garmin InReach Delorme SE on my trip. Other options include the SPOT and personal locator beacons. The InReach sends text messages with your coordinates attached on the Iridium satellite network. Some satellite communicators and PLBs only send out a distress signal that includes your GPS location, but do not allow you to send a text message.

Schrupp, Sandstrom and Norlen all said satellite SOS devices and satellite phones are a good safety tool to have on trail because they allow you to communicate with search and rescue responders when you don't have cell service, and communicate your GPS coordinates. "Any information we can get prior to our crews leaving as far as type of injuries, if they need to be carried, their location, that's great, and helps determine what type of equipment and resources are needed for the rescue situation," Norlen said.

All of these devices require a clear view of the sky to work so they can send and receive signals to and from satellites. Both tree cover and cloud cover can impact their functionality. Before purchasing an SOS device, make sure to research if their satellite network covers your area. Most satellite communicators, aside from PLBs, require a monthly or annual subscription.

The deputies and Norlen aren't fans of the early versions of the SPOT devices, which just sent out a general SOS signal and didn't have texting capabilities. "We get a lot of false calls on those," Schrupp said. "Someone will be playing with it and set it off, not call in that its a false call, and then we have to go in and find them." New versions now have texting capabilities.

On the BRT and Isle Royale, I found having the InReach a personal necessity. The BRT is a true wilderness trail that runs through an area without roads, and motorized craft are not allowed, which means my chance of getting rescued without being able to contact emergency responders was much smaller. I went days without seeing anyone on the BRT. I always bring my InReach on wilderness hikes.

I liked having the option of sending a text rather than a general SOS signal, like the SPOT does. Being able to communicate with emergency responders to give specific information made me feel safer. I am so grateful for the people who are willing to come rescue me, but I never wanted to be the reason they were out there. Every rescue pulls volunteer responders away from their jobs, families, and can involve safety risks for them, too.

You can also get basic weather reports through the InReach. I came to be very accepting of the weather and felt the need for a forecast less and less (Lake Superior often defies weather predictions anyway), but during severe weather it was a great comfort to get a weather report to tell me how long the storm was expected to last.

Like any piece of technology, satellite communicators have some liabilities. Batteries can die. It can take 20 minutes for messages to reach you due to the nature of satellite communication. I've experienced issues with receiving messages with my InReach, which also needed a firmware update halfway into my 75-day trek.

Satellite communicators can be expensive, not just for the hardware, but also for the annual or monthly subscriptions. To me, the cost was worth the peace of mind it gave me and my loved ones back home. Each night I was able to send a message to let them know I was alive and well.

If you're hiking solo, I think these devices can be a valuable tool, but they are not fail proof.

CELL PHONE COVERAGE

From conversation on the SHT Facebook page, it sounds like people with Sprint never have coverage. Verizon customers generally have service except north of Grand Marais and between Crosby-Manitou and Tettegouche state parks; however, signals can be weak and cut out at times. Canadian carriers Rogers and Tbaytel also generally have coverage, since they use Verizon satellites. Toward the northern terminus, it is possible to pick up a Canadian signal, but international roaming charges may apply and can be expensive. Every state park office along the SHT has free wifi.

Most cell phone companies provide a service map on their website. Even if companies list coverage along the SHT, plan on not having it. If you want more security in being able to get medical assistance or rescue on trail, consider investing in a satellite communication device, but even these can have issues if you're in dense tree cover or cloud cover. No communication system is fail-proof in the backwoods. This is one of the risks we have to measure our willingness to accept.

Sometimes your phone can appear to have service, but when you try to call someone, the call either doesn't go through or drops immediately, which can alarm whomever you're trying to reach, said Jo Swanson with the SHTA. "It's much easier to get a text message to send," Swanson said. "A text message either sends or it doesn't," so no one at home is second-guessing whether or not you're OK because of a dropped call.

One of the most magical parts of my thru-hike was putting away my smartphone. For the first time in years, I was forced to be alone with my thoughts for hours on end, day after day. It was really uncomfortable at first, and then became one of my favorites parts of being on trail.

GPS OR APPS

The days of having to bring a separate GPS device are over. There are many smartphone apps that do a great job — Gaia GPS, AllTrails, Guthooks, Avenza and more. These apps work without having cell phone service and on airplane mode. They are much cheaper than handheld GPS devices, but do have some costs if you want more bells and whistles. I wanted the National Geographic maps for my hike, so opted for the $30 annual membership with Gaia GPS. As a safety device, a GPS helps not only by showing you your location in relation to the trail, but also allows you to "drop a pin" on your current location.

"One of the other things we are really promoting in Lake County are apps that you can put on your phone that use the U.S. National Grid. [...] You have to download the app (and relevant maps) while you have cell coverage, but it will continue to operate when you don't have service. It will give you the grid location for where you are. If you do get cell coverage, you can tell a dispatcher your grid location. We can pinpoint you on a map in seconds. That will help our effort significantly," Norlen said.

I used the Gaia GPS app on my iPhone. You have to download maps for the app while you have wifi or cell service for use in the backcountry, and they are big files, akin to downloading a lot of photos. I'd recommend downloading the maps for the next section of trail in each resupply down, then deleting them at your next resupply.

For the SHT, I didn't use the Gaia GPS app much but rather depended on the Kindle-version of the SHTA guide and the SHTA's paper maps. The SHT is so well-marked and maintained, it's really hard to get lost unless you're crossing other trails. On the BRT, the app saved my bacon multiple times because I frequently lost the trail. The GPS app helped me locate my position in relation to the trail, or confirmed that the barely visible tread I was following was indeed the BRT and not an animal trail.

PAPER MAPS AND A COMPASS

Many thru-hikers of well-maintained trails leave paper maps and compasses at home in favor of smartphone apps like Guthooks. I still think maps and a compass are invaluable safety tools. Cell phone batteries die. The green tunnel of trees can block satellite signals.

Orienteering skills increase your safety. There are many good videos on YouTube about how to use a compass, find a bearing, and orient yourself in the backcountry. Outdoor stores like REI and Midwest Mountaineering often offer classes. I went to a Minnesota Orienteering Club (MNOC) event where friendly volunteers taught me the basics. There are several orienteering courses around the Twin Cities metro area as well, for which MNOC provides maps, where you can practice and hone your skills. If you live outside of the Twin Cities metro, search your area for similar orienteering clubs or courses.

WILDERNESS MEDICINE CLASSES

Wilderness medicine classes teach many skills from how to make a splint from on-hand materials to cleaning wounds to knowing when you need to signal for emergency rescue. There are a few respected wilderness medicine class providers like NOLS that offer classes around the country.

I took a two-day Longleaf Wilderness medicine course through Midwest Mountaineering that cost $240. I found it very valuable for improving my general wilderness skills, assessing emergency medical situations, and helping me to decide what level of risk I was willing to take as a solo hiker with my medical supplies.

Wilderness medicine classes are designed for wilderness medical responders and trip guides. The classes don't offer a lot of specific information for solo hikers, but they do teach a general skill set that I used on my hike.

FIRST AID KIT

Most thru-hikers do not bring a big First Aid Kit. I opted not to purchase items like a SAM splint. If I were leading a backpacking group, especially a group in which there were children or people with known health conditions, I would bring a large medical kit.

"Bring bandages, gauze, ace bandage, ointments, creams," Sandstrom said. "You don't need a huge kit to add to your already heavy pack. [Hikers] do have to know their own body, have to know their own ailments. If you have a bum knee, bring a knee wrap."

BUG REPELLANT

So many options exist for bug repellant from Permethrin, used on clothing, tents and packs instead of your skin, to 100 percent DEET. There are little fans that blow tick repellant into the air around you that you can wear on your pack, full body suits of bug netting, and even mosquito repellers that can be attached to fuel canisters.

Ticks and mosquitos carry dangerous diseases. Many hikers use repellant; some don't bother. Jessica Mills, or Dixie, a Triple Crown hiker and vlogger, said she doesn't use DEET because thru-hikers don't shower very often. She thinks reapplying bug spray over and over on your skin without washing it off can be bad for you.

The summer of my hike, conditions were super wet and the bugs were ferocious, the worst I'd ever experienced. The best word to describe the bugs that summer is "apocalyptic." I was putting 100 percent DEET on my skin every hour, and it wasn't working.

I quit using bug repellant on day four of my hike. I switched to wearing a bug net on my head, and my raincoat. It was hot, but I preferred sweating to being driven mad by bugs. At one point the black flies were so thick, one flew straight down my ear canal. After 15 minutes of hiking with a bug scratching around in my ear, I poured water in my ear and drowned it.

Many hikers are a big fan of Permethrin, which is used to treat clothing and gear, and lasts for six washes. It's less toxic to humans than applying DEET directly to your skin. Permethrin is still toxic to the environment, including invertebrates like frogs and lizards, and fish, as well as honey bees, according to the National Pesticide Information Center. I choose not to use pesticides for bug management, but that is a personal decision.

OTHER SAFETY GEAR

There is a lot of other "safety" gear out there — tick keys (for removing ticks), safety whistles, signal mirrors, waterproof match carriers, prepackaged medical kits, space blankets, and more.

My experience: I find most of these specialized safety tools redundant. I don't need a tick key; I have tweezers. I don't need a waterproof match container because I keep an extra lighter in my medical kit as a backup. I don't bring a space blanket because if I'm that cold, I should put my tent up and get in my sleeping bag. I brought a whistle, but by the end of my hike it was so banged up, it didn't make noise anymore. I've since ditched it. My InReach Delorme can send rescuers my exact coordinates, and I can make noise to get rescuers' attention once they're nearby.

Leave no trace

Thru-hikers delight in "trail magic," small acts of kindness from complete strangers that always seem to come at the moment help is most needed. During my trek, examples of trail magic included a clementine left by day hikers outside of my tent while I napped; a ride to a trailhead, saving me miles of roadwalking; and breakfast bought by an older couple thrilled to hear about my adventure and share some tales of their own.

I also love being helpful to others. I wanted to give trail magic, but how? I couldn't lug a 30-pound flat of bottled water to a campsite, or 10 pounds of oranges. It dawned on me: I was giving trail magic to my fellow hikers by following Leave No Trace principles. I picked up all my trash. When another hiker went to bed before me, I tried to keep my noise level down. I walked straight through the mud to reduce my damage to the trail corridor.

Leave No Trace Principles are a set of guidelines to help outdoor recreationists minimize their impact on the wild spaces they love, and be kind to the hiking community. The Seven Principles are: plan ahead and prepare, travel and camp on durable surfaces, dispose of waste properly, leave what you find, minimize campfire impacts, respect wildlife, and be considerate of others, according to the Leave No Trace Center for Outdoor Ethics. The Superior Hiking Trail Association also has a Leave No Trace page on its website. The SHTA also has rules it asks trail users to follow on their Know Before You Go page and their FAQ. Although the SHT often feels remote, like no one else is out there, the SHTA estimates 25,000 people use this trail each year.

The SHTA does maintain the trail and its campsites, but maintenance is expensive and time-intensive. Volunteers adopt campsites and commit to visiting the site twice a year, usually at the beginning and end of hiking season. There is no housekeeping service on the trail; it's up to hikers to keep the SHT and its campsites in good shape day to day.

During Memorial Day weekend in 2017, I volunteered to help clear the trail near Grand Marais. One group discovered someone had thrown a pair of tennis shoes into a campsite latrine. When the trail supervisor was told, he groaned. Any item put into a latrine that isn't toilet paper or human waste has to be pulled out by hand, as signs posted by the SHTA at almost every latrine on the trail explain. When I camped out at Lake Agnes, I rolled out of my tent right on top of someone's else used toilet paper. The latrine was 50 feet away.

When out in the woods far away from trash cans and toilets, managing waste can feel challenging. The effort of limiting our impact on the land and water can be confusing. It's tempting to think, "I'm just one little person, what harm could it do if I just (fill in the blank)?" The harm doesn't come from one person doing something; the harm comes from thousands of people doing the same thing.

The Superior Hiking Trail offers some of the best backpacking and hiking in the state, and is more popular than ever. The increase in users is having a harder impact on the trail as well. Following these Leave No Trace principles will help protect the beauty of the trail for yourself and others for many years to come.

Here are some tricks I've developed over the years to make following Leave No Trace Principles easy. I wish you many magical moments on trail. Please help keep the trail magical for everyone.

Plan and prepare

Know the rules of the trail, and the lands through which it passes. In the case of the SHT, the trail passes through both public and private lands. Hikers not following the SHTA's rules for private land led to the current reroute by Gooseberry State Park when a landowner withdrew permission for the trail to cross his land.

Unlike other long-distance trails, dispersed or stealth camping is not allowed on the Superior Hiking Trail corridor because it passes through so much private land. Camping is only allowed in existing campsites. There are 94 free sites on the trail, plenty for everyone. Stealth camping outside of existing campsites can damage the wilderness corridor along the trail.

Planning ahead helps hikers reduce their impact on the land, and reduces conflicts between people, according to the Center for Outdoor

Ethics. Appropriate planning will prevent stealth camping (barring medical emergencies) and will increase the likelihood that the trail will stay open for everyone. Checking the trail conditions page throughout your hike will alert you to any changes to the trail, or suddenly dangerous areas, as when trails near Carlton Peak were closed in 2018 due to a rock slide.

Stay on the trail;
or embrace the suck(ing mud)

While hiking north out of George Crosby Manitou State Park, I was on the look-out for mud pits reported to be 1-2 feet deep. We'd gotten a lot of rain that year, and the trail felt like one long mud pit, but the idea of fording a river of mud had me in a state of dread. I only found one mud patch that deep. I marveled as my trekking pole sunk 18 inches down. I usually stay right in the center of the tread, even when it's muddy, but I'll admit that I scampered across some very slippery rocks alongside the trail to avoid that quagmire. The SHTA recently launched a trail renewal program and plans to address some of the muddiest areas during the next few years.

On the SHT, conditions are often muddy, especially after heavy rains. Some hikers attempt to keep their feet dry by going around the mud, but generally mud pits aren't one little spot, but rather a large area of muddy ground. Going around one patch just makes the mud patch larger, and your feet still get muddy and wet. Other hikers go further and further out trying to find dry ground. This phenomenon turns an 18-inch tread into a 6-foot-wide swath of mucky, destroyed forest corridor. Embrace nature on nature's terms. Embrace the suck.

TIPS: Having wet feet feels really uncomfortable at first, but you will adjust and barely notice it after a while. Prior to my start date, the Arrowhead region received 5 inches more rain than average, and the trail was one long stretch of mud. I recommend bringing three pairs of socks so you can alternate days to help dry out wet socks. Always keep one pair dry for sleeping so your feet get a break from being wet at night. If "waterproof" boots or shoes get wet, say when you step into a 2-foot deep mud hole, it takes them days to dry out if wet conditions persist. When the trail is wet and muddy, I've found breathable shoes, like trail runners, are best for my feet. In hot, dry conditions, breathable shoes also reduce blisters because my feet are less sweaty.

Please don't put logs across mud pits to cross on as the logs can actually trap water and make the issue worse, according to the SHTA Trail Development Coordinator Jo Swanson.

Dispose of waste properly

Pack it in, pack it out. Many campers burn their trash in the fire ring, which is illegal in Minnesota. The SHTA rules also prohibit burning trash in campfires. "In Minnesota, it is illegal to burn trash of any kind, including paper. Burning trash in a fire grate can release dangerous chemicals into the air and soil, and leaves behind a mess of partially burned items," according to the U.S. Forest Service. Burning left over food also attracts bears and other wildlife to campsites, creating potentially unsafe situations for both people and bears.

TIPS: Most solo thru-hikers won't need more than a gallon zip-lock bag for a week's worth of trash. Bring a couple back-ups in case one breaks. You'll find trash cans along the way, for example in state parks, even when you're not resupplying in town. You will be able to lighten your trash load often, so don't fret about the weight. There are no trash cans at SHT trailheads, and trash shouldn't be left there.

Going to the bathroom without a bathroom

When nature calls and a latrine or toilet isn't close by, dig a 6- to 8-inch cathole 200 feet away from the trail, water or campsites. Mix organic materials like leaf litter into the dirt when you cover your cat hole to help the human waste and toilet paper degrade.

Digging your cathole at least 200 feet away from water sources is crucial if we want to avoid the sad fate of thru-hikers on the Appalachian Trail, where contracting norovirus is so common it seems like a rite of passage. According to the Appalachian Trail Conservancy, most water filters do not filter out viruses. Norovirus lasts one-two days and can cause nausea, vomiting, diarrhea, abdominal cramps, headache, fever, chills and muscle aches. Imagine trying to hike 15 miles while feeling like you have the flu, vomiting, and having explosive diarrhea. Good times!

TIPS: Bring a trowel (or use a tent stake, in a pinch) to dig your cathole. The North Shore has very rocky and rooty soil. Digging a 6-inch hole can be difficult in some places. Dig as far down as you can, and make sure you put a lot of dirt and organic material over your waste in the hole before filling in the hole with dirt. Digging a cat hole is the best option for minimizing the spread of disease and water pollution, and maximizes decomposition.

Wet Wipes are popular among hikers for doing a more thorough cleaning at the end of the day. Wet Wipes should not be thrown in latrines or catholes. They should be packed out.

Tips for the ladies: For proper disposal of urine, a cathole isn't necessary. Just make sure to do your business 200 feet from water sources, campsites and the trail. I keep a small plastic bag inside my toilet paper baggie (a snack ziplock inside the quart-sized zip lock I keep my TP and hand sanitizer in) into which I tuck my used toilet paper so I don't have to bury it. I pack it out. You'll urinate a lot because you'll be drinking a lot of water.

Many female hikers use devices like the P-Style or Shewee, which allows you to urinate while standing up. Some women also hike commando in skirts so they can urinate while standing up. Some women use a "pee rag," a bandana they only use for this purpose. Other female hikers find shaking off to be sufficient, or use leaves they know are safe to come in contact with their skin.

There are several options for managing having your period while thru-hiking. Do not bury your tampons or pads as they take a very long time to decompose, and can be an attractant to animals. Tampons and pads also can't be thrown away in latrines. You have to pack them out. Some female hikers recommend using an empty jerky bag to store used tampons and pads to mask the smell, but I never had any issue with just storing them in my main trash bag. Many female hikers use a menstrual cup like the DivaCup to replace pads and tampons. Menstrual fluid should be dumped into a latrine, into a cat hole 200 feet away from water sources, or packed out. When cleaning a menstrual cup, do it a minimum of 200 feet from water, campsites, and the trail.

The lake is not a bathtub

Bathing with soap contaminates water sources, which can harm wildlife both terrestrial and aquatic, according to the Center for Outdoor Ethics.

I blame the misleading advertisement and labelling of "biodegradable soaps" for the confusion about backcountry washing practices. Soap is slow to degrade in water and can have a lasting impact on water sources. Wash yourself 200 feet away from water sources. I know it seems harmless to take a quick dip in the lake, soap up, and rinse off, but when 500 people do it in the same spot during a single summer, bathing in the lake can make a big impact. If you want to go for a swim, consider first rinsing yourself off 200 feet from the water to remove some of the bug spray, hand sanitizer, etc. coating your skin.

TIPS: Bring some sort of container in which you can store unfiltered water. I use a Sawyer Mini water filter, for which I have two 2-liter collapsible reservoirs that also work great for camp showers. To take a camp bath with soap, follow these steps:

- Place bathing supplies in an area 200 feet away from your water source. When in doubt, go near the latrine which is always a safe distance away from water sources.

- Fill up a couple of reservoirs.

- Go for a swim (or wet yourself down in the water source). Try to enter the water away from where you can tell people usually get water for drinking. You'll see lots of established trails running down to the water.

- Enjoy your swim.

- Go to your bathing location 200 feet away from your water source and soap up. Prioritize the body parts that are likeliest to chafe.

- Rinse off by pouring the water from your reservoirs over you.

- Air dry on a warm rock in the sunshine.

- Revel in your newfound and profound gratitude for your shower at home.

For dishwashing, the center recommends scraping all remaining food particles into your trash bag, then using as little soap as necessary to get the job done. Broadcast the waste water over a large area or pour it into a cathole.

Minimize campfire impacts

Is there anything better than sitting by a softly crackling campfire while dusk falls and a nearby moose cow sings in the woods for a mate? Nope! It's heaven. But with great fires comes great responsibility.

The SHTA requires campfires to be built in provided fire rings at campsites to prevent forest fires, and asks hikers to douse their fires completely when turning into their tents for the night. If conditions are really dry, the U.S. Forest Service or Minnesota Department of Natural Resources will sometimes announce a fire ban. Check with area agencies before your hike to make sure it's legal to have a fire.

Keep your fire reasonable in size, and assess conditions before starting one. Has it been dry and is it a windy night? Conditions may be too risky for a fire. Use dead wood found on the ground that is no larger than your wrist for your fire. Make sure your fire is out and the coals are cold before going to bed. If the coals are too hot to touch, they're too hot to leave unattended.

The last time I was at Lake Agnes, a young man started a fire on the shore of the lake, not in the provided fire grate. When I hiked out the next morning, I saw he'd built his fire on top of what he thought was dirt, but was actually flammable duff, a thick layer of decomposing plant matter, which in this case was mostly pine needles. His fire, which he thought was out, burned down 6 inches into the ground overnight. After I pointed out that his fire was still burning, he doused the fire with water until it stopped smoking completely.

The Ham Lake Fire of 2007 burned 75,000 acres and 150 buildings valued at $10 million; it was the largest forest fire in 80 years in Minnesota. The fire started when a canoeist in the Boundary Waters left his fire unattended, according to the Duluth Tribune. If you're found guilty of setting a forest fire, you can face felony criminal charges and very large fines.

Wildlife and food practices

I set my tent up near Sonju Lake one night before I noticed someone had dumped about 2 pounds of chili mac at the base of a tree a couple feet away. I hadn't noticed it before setting up my tent. Sometimes you cook a huge meal, eat until you're bursting, and still have some leftover. You feel like you can't eat another bite. Please don't dump your food at camp. This will attract rodents, bears and other animals, putting you, other hikers, and the animals at risk. It sucks, but you have to pack your leftovers out. If a bear smells chili mac, comes into camp, and attacks a hiker, that hiker could be badly injured and the bear may be killed by wildlife management. Please don't dump food into latrines for the same reason.

The SHTA requires your food be stored in a way that is inaccessible to bears. Some options are: hanging a bear rope 12 feet off the ground and 6 feet from the trunk of the tree or the nearest branch; storing food in a bear canister; or in an Ursack, a kevlar, bear-proof bag.

TIPS: When you get to camp, you'll have a bunch of "camp chores" to do. Get in the habit of setting up your bear bag before dinner. When the food coma hits, you won't have to spend half an hour looking for a good bear bag branch in the dark.

Storing your food at least 200 feet away from all tents at the campsite is considerate and will minimize the chances that wildlife will disrupt you or your neighbors. I start keeping my eyes peeled for a good tree when I'm within a quarter mile of camp.

To learn more about how to hang your food, a demonstration video by the Center for Outdoor Ethics on the one-branch hang and two-branch hang is available on its website, lnt.org.

Please be considerate of others

The SHTA requires hikers to share campsites. Even if a site feels full, if another group hikes in at dusk, please make room for them. Please share seats around the fire. Please keep your noise level down after camp mates have gone to bed. Some hikers like to sleep in, some are up before dawn. One of my first times on the SHT, I was camped out at the Onion River site with about four other groups. When I woke up around 8 a.m., I crawled out of my tent to an empty campsite. I started laughing because everyone around me had packed up so silently that I'd managed to sleep through their departure. I was impressed and grateful.

TIPS: There are a few popular sites on the SHT near trailheads that tend to attract a lot of hikers on the weekends, and sometimes loud partiers. In my experience, the sites where you're likeliest to run into a loud crowd are Lake Agnes, Section 13, Bear Lake, and Beaver River. If you're thru-hiking and want to avoid the crowds, I'd recommend trying to avoid campsites that are within a half mile of a trailhead on the weekends. Another trick would be to go into town to resupply on the weekend so you're getting off the trail when it's crowded.

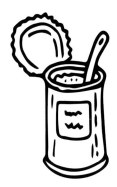

How to resupply

There are two main ways to resupply while thru-hiking: purchase what you need in town, or pack and ship yourself supplies. There are positives and negatives to either system.

You can ship supplies "General Delivery" to post offices along the trail. Several businesses and outfitters also are willing to accept resupply boxes by mail and hold them for thru-hikers.

Trail towns abound on the SHT. You will be able to resupply easily as you go. Food and supplies in resort towns can be more expensive.

If you take medications, eat a special diet, or there are items you'll need on your hike that you're not sure you'll be able to find, you might plan to do a mixture of both. Small town stores can have limited options. Duluth, Two Harbors, Silver Bay, and Grand Marais stock everything stores have in large cities.

A mixture of shipping and purchasing food can help when you are craving ingredients that have a short shelf-life out of the refrigerator, like cheese, more cheese, and did I mention cheese?

I resupplied during my hike by shipping boxes. For a three-month hike, packing resupply boxes was complicated, stressful, and time-consuming, and I ended up buying a lot of food in town anyway. I often couldn't bring myself to eat lemon-dill tuna packets for lunch for the 20th time. I bought in bulk in an attempt to save money, but ended up overspending because I bought more than I needed. If I thru-hike the SHT again, I will not use only resupply boxes for food. Other hikers are trail gourmands who pack themselves amazing resupply boxes and swear by the technique.

Ship supplies

Advantage	Disadvantage
Potential cost-savings buying in bulk and avoiding tourist town prices	May still need to top up supplies in towns
Saves time when resupplying in town	May not accurately predict what you want to eat and buy other food
Ensures meeting specific dietary needs and medication supplies	Easy to under- or over-pack and get stuck with extra weight or not enough food

Purchase in town

Advantage	Disadvantage
Convenience	More time required for shopping
Saves prep time	Pay tourist town prices
Can purchase the types and volumes of food you are craving	Limited selection; may not be able to find what you like
	Heavier if buying fresh ingredients

General shipping instructions

Many hikers use United States Postal Services (USPS) Priority shipping boxes because they cost a flat fee instead of weight-based postage. For international hikers, shipping resupplies once you arrive in the U.S. is recommended. Shipping from the U.S. will save you money, and fuel cannot be shipped internationally.

SHIPPING TO POST OFFICES

Most post offices will hold general delivery packages for 30 days, but the local postmaster can change that to a shorter period. Call each post office ahead of mailing a resupply box to ask how long they're able to hold the package, and if there are any specific ways they'd like the package labelled.

Here is the usual format for addressing general delivery packages:

Your name, General Delivery
Beaver Bay Post Office, 1014 Main St.
Beaver Bay, MN 55601

Hold for SHT thru-hiker
Estimated pickup 8/15/19

Including the street address of the post office isn't necessary as shipping your package general delivery means shipping it to the post office, but it doesn't hurt anything either.

If you end your hike early and won't be picking up your resupply box in person, you can call the post offices and request your boxes be shipped back to you. You will have to pay the postage "COD" (collect on delivery) when you pick up the box.

USING A BOUNCE BOX

Another trick long-distance hikers use to cut down on pack weight and resupply costs are "bounce boxes," which is a general delivery resupply box they "bounce" down the trail by sending it forward to their next resupply location. Follow the same guidelines as with a general delivery box for addressing your bounce box, and then use a new label for your next post office pick up. Common items stored in bounce boxes include: medications, toiletries for bathing in town (shampoo, razor, etc.), sunblock, moleskin, duct tape, replacement journals, foot powder, hand sanitizer, things that will only be worn or used in town (phone and battery chargers, a clean outfit to wear while washing your clothing), replacement Ziplock baggies, and more.

During my five-month hike on the NCT, I used a bounce box for the first few weeks, and found shipping the box more expensive than it was worth. For a shorter hike of three weeks to a month, you'll likely be able to carry most of what you need as far as medical supplies and other hygiene supplies. It was cheaper to purchase what I needed as I went.

SHIPPING TO OUTFITTERS AND BUSINESSES

If shipping to a business or outfitter, always call first, and plan to spend a little money at the business when you pick up your box. It's good manners! Shipping to an outfitter or business where you will need to purchase something anyway, say a fuel canister, can also save you time. There are several businesses along the SHT that are willing to hold resupply boxes, including the Trail Information Office of the Superior Hiking Trail Association. In the resupply list, I note which businesses are willing to hold a resupply box, for what amount of time, and any specific instructions the businesses gave. Please remember, businesses that hold resupply boxes are providing a free service, and doing the hiking community a favor. Businesses that hold resupply boxes are not financially liable if your box never arrives.

SHUTTLE DROP SERVICES

The Superior Hiking Shuttle, Harriet Quarles Shuttle Service and North-shore Shuttles are able to meet you at a trailhead to drop off a resupply box for a fee. Contact the shuttles directly for pricing.

SHIPPING FUEL AND FLAMMABLES

I tried to check with the United States Postal Services about shipping fuel canisters, and even with their help I am not confident in saying whether or not you can. If this is something you really want to do, you'll have to check with your local postmaster. I did learn you cannot ship canisters by Priority Mail, so you will have to pay weight-based postage if it is possible to ship canisters by ground mail. I would recommend not attempting to ship anything flammable (or tobacco and cigarettes) with USPS, FedEx or UPS. Double check with any shipping service before mailing anything that might be considered "hazardous material."

There will be many places to purchase fuel, lighters and matches during your hike. Check local hardware stores, gas stations, gear stores, and outfitters. There are fewer locations where you can recycle fuel canisters. Some outfitters on the North Shore will recycle canisters for you.

Resupply list

Below is a list of resupply options from the southern terminus to the northern terminus. My hope is this list will save you weeks of research time, and be a good resource while you're on trail. This list is exhaustive, but not necessarily comprehensive. If you're wanting to resupply in a location not listed here, reach out to organizations and businesses in the area to see if anyone would be willing to hold a resupply package for you.

One list shows resupply locations in order **NOBO, or northbound**, and the other lists them **SOBO, or southbound.** The charts list the resupply location, amenities in town, distances from the northern and southern trailheads, previous resupply location, and distance from the trail. Each location will include the physical address, phone number, hours of operations, business websites (when available), walking directions from the trail, distances from the southern and northern terminuses, and a list of other nearby businesses and organizations.

If you find any inaccuracies in this list, or think something should be included, please send me an email at thatsawildstory@gmail.com.

Distances are not exact, but close estimates. Trail mileages estimates and walking directions are based on information from the Eighth Edition of the "Guide to the Superior Hiking Trail," Google Maps, Mike Ward's Superior Hiking Trail Distance Calculator, and Kim Fishburn's 2019_Reference_Sheet.pdf in the "Files" tab of the Superior Hiking Trail Facebook group page. Any mathematical mistakes are mine, not theirs. If you spot any math errors, please let me know!

NOBO Superior Hiking Trail Resupply Chart

KEY:

G = Grocery   R = Restaurant

G(L) = Limited grocery or gas station   M = Motel, Hotel or Hostel

G(C) = Co-op   CG = Campground

P = Post Office   B = Resupply Box

L = Laundry   GE = Gear

Location	Trail Mileage	Amenities	Previous Location	Distance from Trail
Duluth Cody St	31*	G, G(C), P, R, M	N/A	2-3 mi
Duluth Rose Garden	40.9	G, G(C), P, L, GE, R, M	11.8 mi	1 block
Duluth Bagley	43.4	G, L	2.5 mi	.5 mi
Duluth Hartley	45.7	G, GE(L), R	2.3 mi	1 mi
Two Harbors	95.7	G, GE, P, L, R, M, B, CG	50 mi	6 mi
Beaver Bay	135.6	G(L), P, L, GE, R, B	39.9 mi	3.1 mi
Silver Bay	139.9	G, GE, P, L, R, M	4.3 mi	3.2 mi
Finland	164.8	G(L), P, B, M	24.9 mi	.3/1.7
Schroeder	196.3	P, CG, R	31.5 mi	1.5mi
Tofte	199	G, GE, R, M	2.4 mi	2.6 mi
Lutsen	215.6	G(L), P, GE(L), M, L, R	16.6 mi	4.5 mi
Cascade Lodge	230	B, M, R	14.4 mi	.2 mi
Grand Marais	246.3	G, P, L, R, M, CG	16.3 mi	1.7 mi
Hungry Hippie	258.7	B, L, M	12.4 mi	1 mi
Hovland	283.7	G(L), P, R	25 mi	3.2 mi
Northern Terminus	298.8**	None	15.1 mi	0 mi

*Includes mileage for hiking to southern terminus from the Wild Valley Road trailhead and back

**Includes mileage for hiking to the northern terminus from the Otter Lake Road trailhead and back

SOBO Superior Hiking Trail Resupply Chart

G = Grocery

G(L) = Limited grocery or gas station

G(C) = Co-op

P = Post Office

L = Laundry

R = Restaurant

M = Motel, Hotel or Hostel

CG = Campground

B = Resupply Box

GE = Gear

Location	Trail Mileage	Amenities	Previous Location	Distance from Trail
Hovland	15.1*	G(L), P, R	N/A	3.2 mi
Hungry Hippie Hostel	39.1	B, L, M	25 mi	1 mi
Grand Marais	51.5	G, P, L, R, M, CG	12.4 mi	1.7 mi
Cascade Lodge	67.2	B, M, R	15.7 mi	.2 mi
Lutsen	82.2	G(L), P, GE(L), M, L, R	15 mi	4.5 mi
Tofte	98.8	G, GE, R, M	16.6 mi	2.7 mi
Schroeder	101.5	P, CG, R	2.7 mi	1.5 mi
Finland	133	G(L), P, B, M	31.5 mi	.3/1.7 mi
Silver Bay	157.9	G, GE, P, L, R, M	24.9 mi	2.8 mi
Beaver Bay	162.2	G(L), P, L, R, B	4.3 mi	1 mi
Two Harbors	202.1	G, GE, P, L, R, M, B, CG	39.9 mi	6 mi
Duluth Hartley	252.1	G, GE(L), R	50 mi	1 mi
Duluth Bagley	254.4	G, L	2.3 mi	.5 mi
Duluth Rose Garden	256.9	G, G(C), P, L, GE, R, M	2.5 mi	1 block
Duluth Cody St	268.7	G, G(C), P, R, M	11.8 mi	2-3 mi
Southern Terminus	299.7*	N/A	29.1 mi	0 mi

*Includes mileage for hiking to the northern terminus from the Otter Lake Road trailhead and back

**Includes mileage for hiking to the southern terminus from the Wild Valley Road trailhead and back

DULUTH

There are many resupply options in Duluth that will be easy to access because of cell service and public transportation. Don't carry an eight-day supply of food like I did through this section. This section of trail is beautiful, and changes frequently in elevation. Keep your food pack light and stay happy.

The section of trail just before the Rose Garden includes the Duluth Lakewalk. You'll pass by dozens of amazing restaurants. Literally, you walk right underneath Fitger's Inn, known for its brewery and great food. This would be a great day to grab a hearty meal in town before you resupply. Many thru-hikers love hiking southbound to Duluth so they can hike themselves right up to a celebratory cold beer.

Duluth Cody Street

Distance from the southern/northern terminuses: 31 mi/268.7 mi

POST OFFICE

U.S. Postal Service

> 2800 W. Michigan St.
> Duluth, MN 55806
> (218) 723-2526 • usps.com

Hours: Monday-Friday 8 a.m.-5 p.m., Saturday 9 a.m.-1 p.m., and Sunday CLOSED

Will hold resupply boxes for 30 days. No lighters or strike-anywhere matches.

Distance from the trail: About 3.1 miles. From intersection of N. 66th Ave. W. and Cody St., follow Cody St. northeast for .8 miles to Memorial Park (N. Central Ave.). Cut straight across park to Grand Avenue and turn left. Follow Grand Ave. for 1.5 miles. Turn right on Carlton Street and follow for .4 miles. Turn left onto W. Michigan Street and follow for .2 miles. Post Office is on your right.

Other nearby organizations and businesses: Stewart's Bikes and Sports, Vintage Italian Pizza, Proctor Federal Credit Union, Tortoise and Hare Footwear, Kwik Trip, Essentia Health-West Duluth Pharmacy, Arby's, Subway, Dairy Queen, Whole Foods Denfeld Co-op, Walgreens, CVS, Perkins, Super 8, Allyndale Motel, McDonald's, Menard's, Super One Foods, and much more.

Other things to know: Any general delivery boxes sent to Duluth will be routed to this post office.

GROCERY

Duluth West Super One Foods

> 5300 Bristol St.
> Duluth, MN 55807
> (218) 628-1965 • superonefoods.com
> **Hours:** Monday-Sunday 6 a.m. to midnight

Distance from trail: 1.1 miles. From intersection of N. 66th Ave. W. and Cody St., go right on Cody St. for half a mile. Turn right on N. 59th St. W. for one block, then left on Wadena St. and follow for a .1 miles. Turn right on N. 57th Ave. W. After .1 miles, 57th turns into Bristol St. after it crosses Grand Ave. Follow for another .2 miles. Super One Foods will be on your right.

Other nearby organizations and businesses: Thrifty White Pharmacy, Menard's, Whole Foods Denfeld Co-op, Western Bank, Spirit Valley Laundromat, Dollar Tree, United States Postal Office, West Duluth Hotel, Domino's Pizza, China King Buffet, Minit Mart, Beaner's Central Coffeehouse, and much more.

Whole Foods Denfeld Co-op

> 4426 Grand Ave.
> Duluth, MN 55807
> (218) 728-0884 ext. 2 • wholefoods.coop
> **Hours:** Monday-Sunday 7 a.m.-9 p.m.

The co-op stocks lots of energy and protein bars, supplements, can do call-ahead orders, and has a great hot bar and deli if you're interested in doing a quick resupply and a meal in the same place.

Distance from trail: 1.4 miles. From intersection of N. 66th Ave. W. and Cody St., follow Cody St. northeast for .8 miles to Memorial Park (N. Central Ave.). When you hit Memorial Park at N. Central Ave., continue straight across park to meet up with Grand Ave., or turn right on Central Ave. to meet up with Grand Ave. At Grand, turn left and follow for half a mile. The co-op will be on your right.

Other nearby organizations and businesses: Super One Foods, Kwik Trip, Arby's, Taco John's, CVS, Walgreens, Menard's, Super 8 Motel.

LAUNDRY

Wash Bucket

> 3004 W. 3rd. St.
> Duluth, MN 55806
> No phone number, currently
> duluthmnlaundromat.com

Hours: Monday-Saturday 8 a.m.-10 p.m. and Sundays 8 a.m.-9 p.m.

Distance from the trail: About 2.7 miles. From intersection of N. 66th Ave. W. and Cody St., follow Cody St. northeast for .8 miles to Memorial Park (N. Central Ave.). When you hit Memorial Park at N. Central Ave., continue straight across park to meet up with Grand Ave., or turn right on Central Ave. to meet up with Grand Ave. At Grand, turn left and follow for half a mile. The laundromat will be on your left.

Other nearby organizations and businesses:
Alano Club (regular Alcoholics Anonymous meetings), A & Dubs.

Duluth Rose Garden

Distance from southern/northern terminuses: 40.9 mi/256.9 mi

GROCERY

Duluth Plaza Super One Foods

> 15 S. 13th Ave. East
> Duluth, MN 55802
> (218) 724-6427 • superonefoods.com

Hours: Monday-Sunday 6 a.m.-10 p.m.

Offers a deli and a patio in the summer with a gorgeous view of Lake Superior if you're looking to grab a meal and resupply in one place.

Distance from trail: One block to the left. From the Duluth Rose Garden, take S. 13th Ave. E. northwest. You will see Super One almost immediately on your left.

Other nearby organizations and businesses: Jimmy John's, Great Harvest Bread Co, Duluth Transit Center, Canal Park Brewing Company, Duluth Running Co., CVS, Walgreens, Trailfitters, and much more.

Whole Foods Co-op

610 E. 4th St.
Duluth, MN 55805
(218) 728-0884 ext. 1 • wholefoods.coop
Hours: Monday-Sunday 7 a.m.-9 p.m.

The bulk section at both the Duluth Co-ops is great for hiking food. You can use your own containers for their bulk section. They have a great selection of trail mix. They also have a deli and hot bar if you want to grab a meal while selecting your trail groceries.

Distance from trail: Right after Fitger's as you're hiking the Lakewalk section of the SHT, you'll see a walkway from the Lakewalk that will bring you up from the lake shore to Superior Street. Take this walkway up to Superior, then turn right and go about .1 miles. Turn left on N. 8th Ave. E. and go .3 miles, then left onto E. 4th St. one block. The co-op will be on your left.

Other nearby organizations and businesses: Uncle Loui's Cafe, Speedway, Va Bene Caffe, Fitger's, St. Luke's Hospital, The Portland Malt Shoppe, The King of Creams, Trailfitters, Maytag Coin Laundry, and more.

LAUNDRY

Maytag Coin Laundry

820 E. 4th St.
Duluth, MN 55805
(651) 775-1914 • maytagcoinlaundry.com
Hours: Monday-Sunday 6 a.m.-10 p.m.

Distance from trail: .5 miles north. From the Lakewalk, take the pedestrian bridge near Fitger's up to Superior St. and turn right. Go one block and turn left on 8th Ave. E. Go eight blocks and turn right on E. 4th St. The laundromat is half a block down on the right.

Other nearby organizations and businesses: Whole Foods Co-op, Uncle Loui's Cafe, Speedway, Va Bene Caffe, Fitger's, St. Luke's Hospital, The Portland Malt Shoppe, The King of Creams, Trailfitters, Super One Foods, and more.

GEAR

Trailfitters

600 E. Superior St.
Duluth, MN 55802
(218) 722-6776 • trailfitters.com

Hours: Monday-Saturday 10 a.m.-9 p.m. and Sunday 11 a.m.-6 p.m.

This gear store caters specifically to backpackers, and its owners and staff are big supporters of the SHT.

Distance from the trail: From the Lakewalk, take the pedestrian bridge near Fitger's up to Superior St. and turn left. Trailfitters is on your left in a couple hundred feet.

Other nearby organizations and businesses: Fitger's, Pickwick Restaurant & Pub, The Portland Malt Shop, Duluth Trading Company, Super One Foods, Whole Foods Co-op, and much more.

Great Lakes Gear Exchange

510 E. 4th St.
Duluth, MN 55805
(218) 481-7270 • greatlakesgearexchange.com

Hours: Tuesday-Friday noon-6 p.m. and Saturday-Sunday 10 a.m.-5 p.m.

Distance from the trail: About 1 mile. From the Lakewalk, take the pedestrian bridge northeast of Sister Cities Park up to Superior St. and go northwest up 1st Ave. E. four blocks to E. 4th St. and turn right, or northeast. Go four blocks and the store will be on your right on the fifth block.

Other nearby organizations and businesses: Speedway, Whole Foods Co-op Hillside, Essentia St. Mary's Medical Center, Trailfitters, Duluth Trading Company, Fitger's, Sheraton Duluth, and much more.

Other things to know: Great Lakes Gear Exchange sells clean, gently used outdoor gear and apparel on consignment in hopes of making outdoor adventure culturally and financially accessible to all while promoting sustainability in the outdoor industry.

Duluth Trading Company

300 E. Superior St.
Duluth, MN 55802
(218) 481-7580 • duluthtrading.com

Hours: Monday-Saturday 10 a.m.-7 p.m. and Sunday 10 a.m.-6 p.m.

Distance from trail: Right after leaving Canal Park, the Lakewalk turns northeast up the shore. Take the first footbridge after this turn to get up to E. Michigan St. and go right one block. The store will be on your left.

Other nearby organizations and businesses: Pizza Lucé, Ragstock, Duluth Coffee Company Cafe, Sheraton Duluth, Mexico Lindo, and much more.

LODGING

Hostel du Nord

> 217 W. 1st St.
> Duluth, MN 55802
> (218) 341-0793 • hosteldunord.com

Price: $45-$90

The hostel has space for 48 people. Each bunk has a privacy curtain, secure storage locker, reading light, and outlet. No pets allowed. Bathrooms are shared. Amenities include a communal space with a shared kitchenette with a microwave and fridge, dining area, and lounge. The hostel has wifi, a Finnish sauna and quiet hours from 10 p.m. to 9 a.m.

Hostel du Nord is willing to hold resupply boxes for thru-hikers who have a reservation at the hostel. Contact the hostel prior to shipping the box to let them know you'll be sending a box, and please include your name somewhere on the box.

Distance from trail: After hiking the Lake Walk, just before the Sister Cities Park and the path bends northeast up Lake Superior, cut across the parking lots to the west to meet up with Lake Ave. Go right two blocks, then left on 1st St. and go three blocks. The hostel will be on your right.

Other nearby organizations and businesses: Toasty's Sandwich Shop, U.S. Bank, Dubh Linn Brew Pub, Starbucks.

Duluth Bagley

Distance from southern/northern terminuses: 43.4 mi/254.4 mi

GROCERY

Duluth Kenwood Super One Foods

> 1316 W. Arrowhead Rd.
> Duluth, MN 55811
> (218) 724-8885 • superonefoods.com

Hours: Monday-Sunday 6 a.m.-10 p.m.

Distance from trail: About .5 miles west of Bagley Nature Center. Before entering the nature center, turn left on E. Buffalo St. then right on Brainerd Ave. and a final left on Arrowhead Road.

Other nearby organizations and businesses: Kenwood Laundromat, Walgreens, Wells Fargo Bank, Arby's, Subway, Holiday, St. Benedict Catholic Church.

LAUNDRY

Kenwood Laundromat

1330 W. Arrowhead Rd.
Duluth, MN 55812
(218) 310-0887 • kenwoodlaundromat.com
Hours: Monday-Sunday 7 a.m.-9 p.m.

Free wifi, on bus routes 11 and 12.

Distance from trail: About .5 miles from the Bagley Nature Center campground at the University of Minnesota Duluth. Follow the trail system in Bagley north to Arrowhead Road, turn left and walk .5 miles. The laundromat is in the Kenwood Shopping Center, right next door to Super One Foods.

Other nearby organizations and businesses: Super One Foods, Walgreens, Wells Fargo Bank, Arby's, Subway, Holiday, St. Benedict Catholic Church.

Other things to know: For NOBO hikers, this is your final opportunity to do laundry until Two Harbors.

Duluth Hartley

Distance from southern/northern terminuses: 45.7 mi/252.1 mi

GROCERY

Duluth Woodland Marketplace Foods

4020 Woodland Ave.
Duluth, MN 55803
(218) 724-4745 • superonefoods.com
Hours: Monday-Sunday 7 a.m.-9 p.m.

Distance from trail: 1 mile. From the Hartley Nature Center, go left on Woodland Ave. and follow for 1 mile. Market will be on your right.

Other nearby organizations and businesses: Cenex gas station, Sammy's Pizza and Restaurant, Zen House restaurant, Woodland Liquors, Denny's Ace Hardware.

GEAR (LIMITED)

Denny's Ace Hardware

> 7 E. Calvary Rd.
> Duluth, MN 55803
> (218) 728-4479 • Denny's Ace Hardware on Facebook

Hours: Monday-Friday 8 a.m.-7 p.m., Saturday 8 a.m.-5:30 p.m., and Sunday 10 a.m.-4 p.m.

TWO HARBORS

Distance from southern/northern terminuses: 95.7 mi/202.1 mi

Two Harbors is a great trail town, and home to the Superior Hiking Trail Association Trail Information Center.

Between Hartley Nature Center in Duluth and Two Harbors, there are no grocery stores. There's about 51 miles of hiking between Hartley and the Reeves Road trailhead on Highway 2 north of Two Harbors. The roadwalk via Highway 2 to Two Harbors is about 6 miles.

To shorten your roadwalk into Two Harbors by 2.5 miles, you could call Arrowhead Transit, 800-862-0175. Arrowhead Transit provides public transportation in Two Harbors for $1.25 a ride Monday-Friday, 9 a.m. to 6 p.m. You can request at pick up at Press Camp Road, which is 3.5 miles south of the Reeves Road trailhead on Highway 2. Arrowhead Transit requires ride requests to be made at least one hour prior to pick up.

POST OFFICE

> Two Harbors Post Office
> 106 Waterfront Dr.
> Two Harbors, MN 55616
> (218) 834-3430 • usps.com

Hours: Monday-Friday 8:30 a.m.-4:30 p.m., Saturday 9-11 a.m. and Sunday CLOSED

Holds resupply boxes for 30 days.

Distance from trail: About 6.1 miles. Head south on Highway 2. Turn right after 5 miles on 5th St. Follow 5th St. for about 1 mile, then turn right on 2nd Ave. and go one block. Turn left on 6th St. The post office will be on the left.

Other nearby organizations and businesses: Granite Gear, Super One, Burlington Bay Campground, Holiday, Judy's Cafe, Bay Breeze Laundry, Seagren's Hardware Store, Castle Danger Brewery, Voyageur Motel, Viking Motel, and more.

RESUPPLY BOX

Superior Hiking Trail Association Trail Information Center

618 1st Ave.
Two Harbors, MN 55616
(218) 834-2700 • superiorhiking.org
Hours: Monday, Thursday and Friday, 10 a.m.-4:30 p.m.

The Trail Information Center is able to hold resupply boxes for hikers. Contact the SHTA at info@superiorhiking.org to arrange. If hikers need to pick up a box on a weekend or anytime the SHTA isn't open, the packages will be left in an unsecured location where they can be picked up 24/7. They have trail maps, the guide, and the most up-to-date trail conditions information. Plus, it's really fun to stop in and say hello to the folks who make this trail happen! Although the Trail Information Center has limited hours, the SHTA is able to leave the box outside in a safe location, but hikers need to call ahead and speak with an actual person (not just leave a voicemail) to arrange an after-hours pick-up.

Distance from the trail: About 5.8 miles. Head south on Highway 2. After about 4.5 miles, turn right on 23rd Ave. Turn left on 7th Ave. and go .2 miles. At 20th Ave., 7th St. turns into Paul Antonich Dr., continue straight for .3 miles. At 16th Ave., Paul Antonich Dr. turns into 8th St. Continue straight for .6 miles to 7th Ave. (Highway 61). The Trail Information Center will be to your left on the corner of 8th St. and 7th Ave.

Other nearby organizations and businesses: Granite Gear, Post Office, Burlington Bay Campground, Holiday, Judy's Cafe, Bay Breeze Laundry, Lakeview Pharmacy, Seagren's Hardware Store, Castle Danger Brewery, Voyageur Motel, Viking Motel, and more.

GROCERY

Two Harbors Super One Foods

802 11th St.

Two Harbors, MN 55616

(218) 834-5651 • superonefoods.com

Hours: Monday-Sunday 6 a.m.-10 p.m.

Distance from trail: About 6 miles. Head south on Highway 2. After about 4.5 miles, turn right on 23rd Ave. Turn left on 7th Ave. then right on 20th Ave., which turns into 11th Street, which you follow right to Super One.

Other nearby organizations and businesses: Granite Gear, Post Office, Burlington Bay Campground, Holiday, Judy's Cafe, Bay Breeze Laundry, Lakeview Pharmacy, Seagren's Hardware Store, Castle Danger Brewery, Voyageur Motel, Viking Motel, and more.

LAUNDRY

Bay Breeze Laundry

1303 7th Ave.

Two Harbors, MN 55616

(218) 834-6106 • Bay Breeze Laundry on Facebook

Hours: Monday-Sunday 7:30 a.m.-10 p.m.

Distance from trail: About 7.3 miles. Head south on Highway 2. After about 4.5 miles, turn right on 23rd Ave. Turn left on 7th Ave. then right on 20th Ave., which turns into 11th Street. Follow 11th all the way to 7th St. (also Highway 61) and take a right. The laundry will be on your right in about half a mile.

Other nearby organizations and businesses: Super One Foods, Granite Gear, Post Office, Burlington Bay Campground, Holiday, Judy's Cafe, Lakeview Pharmacy, Seagren's Hardware Store, Castle Danger Brewery, Voyageur Motel, Viking Motel, and more.

LODGING

Voyageur Motel

1227 7th Ave. (Highway 61)

Two Harbors, MN 55616

(218) 834-3644 • Voyageur Motel on Facebook

Price: Changes depending on season and day of the week. Call for pricing. Owners say they have the lowest prices in town.

Free wifi, close to the laundromat and grocery store. Do North Pizza also delivers to the motel, free coffee in office. Dog-friendly, but one-time $10 additional charge.

Distance from trail: About 6.3 miles. Head south on Highway 2. After about 4.5 miles, turn right on 23rd Ave. Turn left on 7th Ave. then right on 20th Ave., which turns into 11th Street. Follow 11th all the way to 7th St. (also Highway 61) and take a right. The motel will be on your right in .2 miles.

Other nearby organizations and businesses: Super One Foods, Granite Gear, Post Office, Burlington Bay Campground, Holiday, Judy's Cafe, Lakeview Pharmacy, Seagren's Hardware Store, Castle Danger Brewery, and more.

Viking Motel

1429 7th Ave.
Two Harbors, MN 55616
(218) 834-2645

Price: Call for pricing

Wifi, dog-friendly, close to the laundromat and grocery store. Do North Pizza also delivers to the motel.

Distance from trail: About 6.4 miles. Head south on Highway 2. After about 4.5 miles, turn right on 23rd Ave. Turn left on 7th Ave. then right on 20th Ave., which turns into 11th Street. Follow 11th all the way to 7th St. (also Highway 61) and take a right. The motel will be on your right in about .3 miles.

Other nearby organizations and businesses: Super One Foods, Granite Gear, Post Office, Burlington Bay Campground, Holiday, Judy's Cafe, Lakeview Pharmacy, Seagren's Hardware Store, Castle Danger Brewery, and more.

GEAR

Granite Gear

2312 10th St.
Two Harbors, MN 55616
(218) 834-6157 • granitegear.com

Hours: Monday-Friday 9 a.m.-4:30 p.m., CLOSED Saturday and Sunday

Sells packs and pack accessories.

Distance from trail: About 5 miles. From the Reeves Road trailhead parking lot, turn right on Highway 2 and go 4.3 miles. Turn right on

23rd. Ave. and continue when road changes to Lake County 200 S. for .3 miles. Turn right on 10th St. and the Granite Gear storefront will be on your right.

Other nearby organizations and businesses: Super One Foods, Post Office, Bay Breeze Laundry, Burlington Bay Campground, Holiday, Judy's Cafe, Lakeview Pharmacy, Seagren's Hardware Store, Castle Danger Brewery, Voyageur Motel, Viking Motel, and more.

Seagren's Hardware Store

610 1st Ave.
Two Harbors, MN 55616
(218) 834-2222 • ww3.truevalue.com/seagrenstruevalue
Hours: Monday-Friday 8 a.m.-5:30 p.m., Saturday 8 a.m.-5 p.m., and Sunday 10 a.m.-3 p.m.

If you are having a gear emergency, and can't make it to the store by closing, Seagren's is willing to stay open a bit later for you. They carry a lot of camping gear and supplies, including fuel: canisters, propane, alcohol and Esbit tabs.

Distance from trail: About 6 miles. From the Reeves Road trailhead parking lot, turn right on Highway 2 and go 5 miles to 5th Street. Turn right and go west .1 miles. Where 5th Street meets 13th Avenue, it turns south. Follow 5th for another .8 miles. Turn right on 1st Avenue and go one block. Seagren's will be on the left.

Other nearby organizations and businesses: Super One Foods, Post Office, Bay Breeze Laundry, Burlington Bay Campground, Holiday, Judy's Cafe, Lakeview Pharmacy, Castle Danger Brewery, Voyageur Motel, Viking Motel, and more.

BEAVER BAY

Distance from southern/northern terminuses: 135.6 mi/162.2 mi

There is no grocery store in Beaver Bay, but there is a convenience store, a post office, and a laundromat. Most hikers opt to stop in Silver Bay instead since it is one of the best trail towns on the SHT and just a couple miles away.

There are two ways to walk into Beaver Bay, one that avoids road walking by using the Cove Point Loop spurs and the Gitchi Gami State Trail, and the other by a very manageable .8-mile roadwalk southeast from Lax Lake Road Trailhead.

Spur Trail: The distance to town along the spur trails is about 3 miles if following the western spur of the Cove Point Loop (the first spur when traveling northbound), and 2.5 miles if following the eastern spur (the first when traveling southbound). The Cove Point Loop spurs form a "lollipop" meaning they join into a single spur trail before you reach Highway 61. When hikers meet up with the Gitchi Gami State Trail, turn left and the paved bike trail will take you to the intersection of Slater Drive and Highway 61 in Beaver Bay.

Roadwalk: For the roadwalk, turn southeast and go .8 miles along Lax Lake Road.

POST OFFICE

Beaver Bay Post Office

1014 Main St.
Beaver Bay, MN 55601
(218) 226-4129 • usps.com

Hours: Monday-Friday 12:30-4:30 p.m., Saturday 9-10 a.m., CLOSED Sunday

Will hold resupply boxes for 30 days.

Distance from trail: By Cove Point Loop Spurs: About 3 miles if following the western spur, and 2.5 miles if following the eastern. Once at the intersection of Slater Drive and Highway 61, go right on 61/Main Street for one block. The post office will be on your right.

By roadwalk, about 1 mile. Follow Lax Lake Road for .6 miles, then turn right at Old Towne Road and go about .3 miles to Main Street. The post office will be kitty corner across Main Street.

*The Cove Point spur is a "lollipop." The eastern and western spurs form a "Y" shape and join into a single trail before you reach Highway 61.

Other nearby organizations and businesses: Red Raven North, Holiday, Mother Load Laundry, Mobil, Beaver Bay Fire Department, Lemon Wolf Cafe, and more.

GROCERY

Holiday

1015 Main St.
Beaver Bay, MN 55601
(218) 226-3227 • holidaystationstores.com
Hours: Monday-Sunday 5 a.m.-11 p.m.

Small selection of camping gear.

Distance from trail: By Cove Point Loop Spurs: About 3 miles if following the western spur, and 2.5 miles if following the eastern. Once at the intersection of Slater Drive and Highway 61, go right on 61/Main Street for one block. The store will be on your left.

By roadwalk, about 1 mile. Follow Lax Lake Road for .6 miles, then turn right at Old Towne Road and go about .3 miles to Main Street. Turn left. The store will be on your left.

Other nearby organizations and businesses: Post Office, Red Raven North, Mother Load Laundry, Mobil, Beaver Bay Fire Department, Lemon Wolf Cafe, and more.

LAUNDRY

The Mother Load Laundry

309 Old Towne Rd.
Beaver Bay, MN 55601
(218) 226-3936 • The Mother Load Laundry LLC on Facebook
Hours: Open 24 hours

Located behind Holiday. Drop-off service available.

Distance from trail: By Cove Point Loop Spurs: About 3 miles if following the western spur, and 2.5 miles if following the eastern. Once at the intersection of Slater Drive and Highway 61, go right on 61/Main Street for one block. The laundromat is behind the Holiday on your left.

By roadwalk, about 1 mile. Follow Lax Lake Road for .6 miles, then turn right at Old Towne Road and go about .3 miles to Main Street. Turn left. The laundromat is behind Holiday on your left.

Other nearby organizations and businesses: Post Office, Red Raven North, Holiday, Mobil, Beaver Bay Fire Department, Lemon Wolf Cafe, and more.

LODGING/RESUPPLY BOX

Red Raven North

1017 Main St.
Beaver Bay, MN 55601
(218) 830-0955
Hours: Call for hours

Price: $60-$149. Rooms are listed on AirBnb as "Raven North: Nest 2" and Raven North: Nest 6." Self-check in, keyless entry offered.

Formerly Camp 61, the new owners of Red Raven North are big hikers and even got married on the Superior Hiking Trail. They are willing to hold resupply boxes for thru-hikers. They will also be adding a coffee shop, bike rentals, and a retail space with supplies hikers need, owner Julie McGinnis said.

Distance from trail: By Cove Point Loop Spurs: About 3 miles if following the western spur, and 2.5 miles if following the eastern. Once at the intersection of Slater Drive and Highway 61, go right on 61/Main Street for one block. Red Raven North will be on your left.

By roadwalk, about 1 mile. Follow Lax Lake Road for .6 miles, then turn right at Old Towne Road and go about .2 miles. Red Raven North will be on your right before you reach Highway 61.

Other nearby organizations and businesses: Post Office, Holiday, Mother Load Laundry, Mobil, Beaver Bay Fire Department, Lemon Wolf Cafe, and more.

Cove Point Lodge

4616 Hwy 61
Beaver Bay, MN 55601
(218) 226-3221 • covepointlodge.com

Hours: 24 hours a day

Price: $169-$250. When booking a room in advance, Cove Point Lodge does require a two-night minimum stay, but if there is an opening, walk-ins can get a room for one night.

Cove Point Lodge is able to hold resupply boxes. The managers are avid hikers and love being supportive to hikers. They ask thru-hikers to please contact the lodge before shipping a box, and to make sure your name is on the box somewhere. They are held at the front desk. It is also possible to leave a vehicle parked long-term at the lodge, except during their busy seasons in July and October.

Cove Point Lodge also has two restaurants. The restaurant in the lodge is more formal, plated dinners. At top of the hill, there is a more casual pizza and sandwich shop, but both restaurants do to-go orders.

Distance from trail: About 3 miles if following the western arm of the Cove Point Loop spur trail, and 2.5 if following the eastern arm. The lodge is located at the end of the spur.

Other nearby organizations and businesses: Post office, Red Raven North, Holiday, Lemon Wolf Cafe and more.

SILVER BAY

Distance from southern/northern terminuses: 139.9 mi/157.9 mi

If you can resupply and take a rest day in Silver Bay, do it. This mining town offers a great grocery store called Zup's Food Market, a laundromat, great burgers at Northwoods Family Grille, and a reasonably priced accommodations at the Mariner Motel. All are in close proximity to the trail.

Two options exist for walking into town: a quick 1.6-mile roadwalk or a longer 2.7- or 3.2-mile hike down the beautiful Bean and Bear Lakes spur trail, also known as the Twin Lakes Loop.

Roadwalk: From the Penn Boulevard Trailhead, turn east on Penn Boulevard and go 1.6 miles to the town business center.

Spur Trail: The Twin Lakes spurs are a "lollipop," meaning the eastern and western spurs form a "Y" shape and join into a single trail before you reach the Bay Area Historical Society Parking lot. If you take the western spur (the first spur if you're traveling northbound), it is about 3.2 miles. If you take the eastern spur (the first spur if traveling south), the hike is about 2.7 miles.

POST OFFICE

Silver Bay Post Office

13 Shopping Center Rd.
Silver Bay, MN 55614
(218) 226-3700 • usps.com

Hours: Monday-Friday 8 a.m.-12:30 p.m. and 1:30-4:30 p.m., CLOSED Saturday and Sunday

Can't accept UPS packages, only packages sent through the United States Postal Service. Please write your estimated date of arrival on the box. Will hold resupply boxes for 30 days.

Distance from trail: By roadwalk, the post office is 1.6 miles. Follow Penn Boulevard for 1.5 miles east, then turn left at Shopping Center Road. The post office will be on your left. By spur trail, the post office is 3.2 miles by the western spur, and 2.7 miles by the eastern spur. From the Historical Society parking lot, turn right on Davis Drive and go one block and turn left on Banks Boulevard. Go one block to Shopping Center Road and turn left. The post office is in the shopping center to your right.

Other nearby organizations and businesses: Julie's True Value, Zup's Food Market, Northwoods Family Grille, Zupancich Brothers Big Dollar, Bri-Esa's Convenience Store, The Lake Bank, Silver Bay Municipal Liquor, Jimmy's Pizza, J&H Auto Repair (has laundromat) and more.

GROCERY

Zup's Food Market

> 3 Shopping Center
> Silver Bay, MN 55614
> (218) 226-4161 • zups.com

Hours: Summer hours: Monday-Saturday 8 a.m.-8 p.m., Sunday 9 a.m.-4 p.m.

Homemade jerky, and homemade sausages.

Distance from trail: By roadwalk, Zup's is 1.6 miles. Follow Penn Boulevard for 1.5 miles east, then turn left at Shopping Center Road. The store will be on your left. By spur trail, Zup's is 3.2 miles by the western spur, and 2.7 miles by the eastern spur. From the Historical Society parking lot, turn right on Davis Drive and go one block and turn left on Banks Boulevard. Go one block to Shopping Center Road and turn left. Zup's is in the shopping center to your right.

Other nearby organizations and businesses: Julie's True Value, United States Post Office, Northwoods Family Grille, Zupancich Brothers Big Dollar, Bri-Esa's Convenience Store, The Lake Bank, Silver Bay Municipal Liquor, Jimmy's Pizza, J&H Auto Repair (laundromat) and more.

LAUNDRY

J&H Auto Repair and Towing

> 91 Outer Dr.,
> Silver Bay, MN 55614
> (218) 226-4447 • jh-towing-recovery.business.site

Hours: Open 24 hours a day

The laundromat is on the side of the auto shop and does not have its own business name.

Distance from trail: By roadwalk, J&H's is 1.6 miles. Follow Penn Boulevard for 1.6 miles east. The laundromat will be on your right at the intersection with Shopping Center Road. By spur trail, J&H's is 3.2 miles by the western spur, and 2.7 miles by the eastern spur. From the Historical Society parking lot, cross the parking lot to the far driveway to get to

Outer Drive and turn right. Go one block. J&H Auto will be on your left after the intersection of City Shop Road.

Other nearby organizations and businesses: Zup's Food Market, Julie's True Value, United States Post Office, Northwoods Family Grille, Zupancich Brothers Big Dollar, Bri-Esa's Convenience Store, The Lake Bank, Silver Bay Municipal Liquor, Jimmy's Pizza, and more.

LODGING

Mariner Motel

> 46 Outer Dr.
> Silver Bay, MN 55614
> (218) 226-4488

Price: Call for prices

> *Allows dogs for extra charge
> *Offers discount if paying in cash

The owner of the Mariner Motel is infamous among SHT hikers and Yelp reviewers, due to his mercurial disposition. Some people have had great interactions with him, others dislike him. I found the motel reasonable in cost, very clean, and enjoyed my stay. My interaction with the owner, Wes, was memorable and funny. He teased me a lot about my "extreme" endeavor of thru-hiking the trail.

Distance from trail: By roadwalk, the Mariner Motel is 2.1 miles. Follow Penn Boulevard for 2.1 miles east. The motel will be on your left just before Highway 61. By spur trail, the motel is 3.3 miles by the western spur, and 2.7 miles by the eastern spur. From the Historical Society parking lot, cross the parking lot to the far driveway to get to Outer Drive and turn left. From the Historical Society parking lot, cross the parking lot to the far driveway to get to Outer Drive and turn left. Follow Outer Drive for .5 miles. The motel will be on your left.

Other nearby organizations and businesses: Zup's Food Market, J&H Auto (laundromat), Julie's True Value, United States Post Office, Northwoods Family Grille, Zupancich Brothers Big Dollar, Bri-Esa's Convenience Store, The Lake Bank, Silver Bay Municipal Liquor, Jimmy's Pizza, and more.

AmericInn

150 Mensing Dr.
Silver Bay, MN 55614
(218) 226-4300 • wyndhamhotels.com

Price: Call for pricing

AmericInn allows thru-hikers to shower for $5 even if they aren't staying at the hotel. You can also pay a small fee to take a dip in their pool. The manager at the hotel often goes for hikes on the SHT and is very supportive of people using the trail. Employees at the hotel have even been known to give hikers a free ride to nearby trailheads.

Distance from trail: By roadwalk, AmericInn is 2.9 miles from the Penn Boulevard Trailhead. Head east down the boulevard 1.1 miles, continue onto Outer Drive another mile, turn left or northeast at Highway 61 and go .6 miles. The hotel will be on your right. By spur trail, the hotel is about 3.3 miles. If traveling NOBO, it's the first spur after the Penn Creek campsite. About 2.7 miles down the eastern spur* of the Bean and Bear Lakes trail if traveling SOBO. The eastern spur is about .1 miles before the Bear Lake campsite. The spur trail ends at the Bay Area Historical Society parking lot. From the lot, AmericInn is another 1.3 miles. Walk across the parking lot to the far drive and take a left on Outer Dr. Follow Outer Dr. for .5 miles to Highway 61 and turn left. Go another .4 miles to Mensing Dr. and turn right. The hotel will be visible at this point. Follow Mensing when it curves to the left. The hotel will be straight ahead.

*The Twin Lakes spur is a "lollipop." The eastern and western spurs form a "Y" shape and join into a single trail before you reach the Bay Area Historical Society parking lot.

Other nearby organizations and businesses: Zup's Food Market, J&H Auto (Laundry), Julie's True Value, United States Post Office, Northwoods Family Grille, Zupancich Brothers Big Dollar, Bri-Esa's Convenience Store, The Lake Bank, Silver Bay Municipal Liquor, Jimmy's Pizza, and more.

FINLAND

Distance from southern/northern terminuses: 164.8 mi/133 mi

Finland is another great place to resupply. The Clair Nelson Center (formerly known as the Finland Community Center) is a short .3 miles down a spur trail from the main SHT and is willing to hold resupply packages for hikers. The staff are incredibly supportive of hikers and, if you're lucky, you'll pass by during a meeting of the area craft club and be gifted some fresh watermelon and cherries like me. The center hosts a Farmers Market from 5-6:30 p.m. on Thursday nights starting mid-June until early October. Finland also has a small co-op grocery that is able to accept resupply boxes and a post office.

POST OFFICE

Finland Post Office

6638 Highway 1
Finland, MN 55603
(218) 353-7318 • usps.com

Hours: Monday-Friday 8 a.m. to noon, Saturday 10-11 a.m., CLOSED Sunday

Able to hold resupply boxes for 30 days.

Distance from trail: About 1.8 miles from the spur trail. Head southwest (toward Finland Community Center) on Highway 7 or Cramer Road for 1 mile, then turn left on Highway 1 for another .4 miles. The post office will be on your left directly behind the Finland Cooperative.

Other nearby organizations and businesses: Clair Nelson Center, Mobil, Finland Cooperative, West Branch Bar and Grill, Our Place.

RESUPPLY BOX

Clair Nelson Center

6866 Cramer Rd.
Finland, MN 55603
(218) 353-0300 • Clair Nelson Center Facebook page

Hours: Monday 6-8 p.m., Tuesday 10 a.m.-4 p.m. and 6-8 p.m., Wednesday 10 a.m.-4 p.m. and 6-8 p.m., Thursday CLOSED, Friday 10 a.m.-4 p.m., Saturday and Sunday CLOSED

Special instructions: Please contact the Finland Community Center before sending a resupply package. When the center is closed, staff respond quickly when messaged through Facebook Messenger and are incredibly supportive of SHT thru-hikers. If you know you'll be arriving for your resupply package when the center is closed, they will put your box in a corner of the front entryway, which is open 24 hours a day. The center needs to know your approximate pick-up date, and asks hikers to ship through FedEx or UPS, because if they come to the post office, the center may not get them. Please include an arrival date, and disposal date on the package. If a hiker's plans change after they've shipped a box, the center asks to be notified.

Distance from trail: Immediately off of .3-mile spur trail of main SHT.

Other nearby organizations and businesses: Finland Cooperative, Mobil, Post Office, West Branch Bar and Grill, Our Place.

GROCERY

Finland Cooperative

6648 Highway 1
Finland, MN 55603
(218) 353-7389 • finlandcoop.com

Hours: Monday-Sunday 6 a.m.-9 p.m.

Willing to hold resupply boxes. They ask you to make sure the box has your name on it, and your estimated pickup date. The co-op stocks many things you might need mid-hike: fuel (propane fuel, isopropyl butane fuel, and white gas fuel canisters), hardware, groceries and first-aid products.

Distance from trail: About 1.8 miles from the spur trail. Head southwest (toward Finland Community Center) on Highway 7 or Cramer Road for 1 mile, then turn left on Highway 1 for another .4 miles. The co-op will be on your left.

Other nearby organizations and businesses: Clair Nelson Center, Mobil, Post Office, West Branch Bar and Grill, Our Place.

SCHROEDER

Distance from southern/northern terminuses: 196.3 mi/101.5 mi

Schroeder offers limited resupply options: a post office, resort, and great bakery. The small community can be reached by hiking down a short 1.5 mile spur trail along the Cross River.

POST OFFICE

Schroeder Post Office

> 7940 W. Highway 61
> Schroeder, MN 55613
> (218) 663-7568 • usps.com

Hours: Monday-Friday 12:30-4:30 p.m. and Saturday 8-10 a.m. Sunday CLOSED

The standard hold time for resupply boxes is 15 days. On the box, please give an expected arrival date. If your arrival date is later than the standard 15 days, they will hold the box until your date.

Distance from trail: About half a mile from the spur trail. Once you reach the Skou Road trailhead, follow Skou Road down to Highway 61 and turn right. Walk another quarter mile. The post office, Lamb's Resort, and the bakery are all on Lake Superior side of Highway 61. There are sidewalks along Highway 61 here, so there is no dangerous road walk.

Other nearby organizations and businesses: Lamb's Resort, Schroeder Baking Co., Cross River Heritage Center.

LODGING

Lamb's Resort

> 19 Lamb's Way
> Schroeder, MN 55613
> (218) 663-7292 • lambsresort.com

Open: May through October

Price: $41.95 plus tax for campsites.

Lamb's is willing to hold resupply boxes for thru-hikers.

*Pets are welcome but must be registered ($10 exta fee).

*If there is more than one tent at the site in which an adult is sleeping, there is an additional $10 charge. There is no additional charge if only children are sleeping in the tent.

*Wifi available near office and arcade building.

OTHER

Schroeder Baking Company

19 Lamb's Way

Schroeder, MN 55613

(218) 663-7331 • Schroeder Baking Company Facebook page

Hours: Only open seasonally, spring to fall, and hours vary by season. Check their Facebook page for the most up-to-date information.

I took a full rest day at Lamb's, and just to tell you how great this little bakery is, I ate there five times in less than 24 hours. They offer amazing pastries, great coffee, but also pizza, sandwiches and other snacks. I loved my easy, restful, donut-filled resupply in Schroeder. The bakery also has free wifi.

TOFTE

Distance from southern/northern terminuses: 199 mi/98.8 mi

A few miles down the trail from Schroeder, Tofte offers resupply options and other amenities including a post office, general store, and an outfitter that sells outdoor gear.

POST OFFICE

Tofte Post Office

7223 Tofte Park Rd.

Tofte, MN 55615

(218) 663-7985 • usps.com

Hours: Monday-Friday 8-11 a.m. and 1-4 p.m., and Saturday 8:30-9:30 a.m.

Holds resupply boxes for 30 days. Please write your estimated date of arrival on the box.

Distance from the trail: About 2.2 miles northeast from Temperance River State Park, following the Gitchi Gami State Trail (a paved bike trail) out of the park. The Superior Hiking Trail crosses the Temperance River on a metal bridge, which is also the bike trail. Instead of following the SHT back up the river, go straight on the Gitchi Gami for 1.5 miles. When you reach Highway 61, cross 61 and take Tofte Park Road about half a mile to avoid a highway road walk. The post office will be on your left.

Alternate route: From the Britton Peak trailhead, the post office is about 2.7 miles southeast down the Sawbill Trail. Turn left out of the trailhead parking lot onto Sawbill Trail. When you reach Highway 61, turn right and walk a half mile down 61 to Tofte Park Road and turn left. The post office will be on your right.

Other nearby businesses and organizations: Coho Cafe, North Shore Commercial Fishing Museum, Bluefin Grill, Bluefin Bay on Lake Superior (hotel), Sawtooth Outfitters, Holiday, Tofte Ranger Station for Superior National Forest, Zoar Lutheran Church, Waves of Lake Superior Spa, Grand Marais State Bank, Waters Edge Trading Company.

GROCERY

Tofte General Store and Bottle Shop

> 7125 W. Highway 61
> Tofte, MN 55615
> (218) 663-7288 • Tofte General Store and Bottle Shop Facebook page

Hours: Monday-Saturday 8 a.m.-7 p.m. and Sunday 8 a.m.-6 p.m.

Groceries, and camping fuel: kerosene and propane only. The Bottle Shop sells liquor, beer and wine.

Distance from trail: About 2.6 miles northeast from Temperance River State Park, following the Gitchi Gami State Trail (a paved bike trail) out of the park. The Superior Hiking Trail crosses the Temperance River on a metal bridge, which is also the bike trail. Instead of following the SHT back up the river, go straight on the Gitchi Gami for 1.5 miles. When you reach Highway 61, cross 61 and take Tofte Park Road about half a mile, and then turn right on 61 for the final third of a mile.

Alternate route: From the Britton Peak Trailhead, the store is about 2.4 miles. Turn left out of the trailhead parking lot and follow the Sawbill Trail into town. At the intersection with Highway 61, the store will be on your left.

Other nearby businesses and organizations: Coho Cafe, North Shore Commercial Fishing Museum, Bluefin Grill, Bluefin Bay on Lake Superior (hotel), Sawtooth Outfitters, Holiday gas station, Tofte Ranger Station for Superior National Forest, Zoar Lutheran Church, Waves of Lake Superior Spa, Grand Marais State Bank, Waters Edge Trading Company.

Holiday

7235 W. Highway 61
Tofte, MN 55615
(218) 663-7882 • holidaystationstores.com

Hours: Monday-Sunday 6 a.m.-10 p.m.

Full convenience store, and sporting goods like sleeping bags, propane and butane fuel canisters, and other camping gear. Has HEET for alcohol stoves.

Distance from the trail: About 2 miles northeast from Temperance River State Park, following the Gitchi Gami State Trail (a paved bike trail) out of the park. The Superior Hiking Trail crosses the Temperance River on a metal bridge, which is also the bike trail. Instead of following the SHT back up the river, go straight on the biking trail for 1.5 miles. When you reach Highway 61, cross 61 and take Tofte Park Road about a third of a mile, then turn left on Netland Rd. When you reach Highway 61, the gas station will be directly across the highway.

Alternate route: The store is about 2.7 miles southeast from the Britton Peak trailhead down Sawbill Trail. At Highway 61 turn right, and walk about a half mile down 61. The store will be on your right.

Other nearby businesses and organizations: Tofte General Store, Coho Cafe, North Shore Commercial Fishing Museum, Bluefin Grill, Bluefin Bay on Lake Superior (hotel), Sawtooth Outfitters, Tofte Ranger Station for Superior National Forest, Zoar Lutheran Church, Waves of Lake Superior Spa, Grand Marais State Bank, Waters Edge Trading Company.

GEAR

Sawtooth Outfitters

7213 Highway 61
Tofte, MN 55615
(218) 663-7643 • sawtoothoutfitters.com

Hours: The store is typically open the first weekend in May through the Friday of Memorial weekend 8 a.m.-6 p.m. Monday-Sunday, Memorial Day weekend through Labor Day weekend 7 a.m.-7 p.m. Monday-Sunday. After Labor Day, they are open 8 a.m.-6 p.m. Monday-Sunday through late October. The store closes until mid December and reopens mid-December through April 8 a.m.-6 p.m. Monday-Sunday.

Sawtooth stocks all needed camping and backpacking supplies, except long-distance backpacks. They do stock repair items for tents and packs. For fuel, they stock isobutane stove, liquid fuel, and propane. The also rent gear if you have a failure and don't want to invest in a new piece of gear. Sawtooth is also willing to hold resupply boxes. They ask that thru-hikers call before mailing a package, and ask that the box have your name, and an estimated pickup date. Sawtooth will hold boxes up to two weeks after that date in case you are delayed.

Distance from the trail: About 2.2 miles northeast from Temperance River State Park, following the Gitchi Gami State Trail (a paved bike trail) out of the park. The Superior Hiking Trail crosses the Temperance River on a metal bridge, which is also the bike trail. Instead of following the SHT back up the river, go straight on the Gitchi Gami for 1.5 miles. When you reach Highway 61, cross 61 and take Tofte Park Road about half a mile to avoid a highway road walk. Turn left onto Tofte Homestead Dr. and cross back over Highway 61. The outfitter will be directly in front of you.

Alternate route: The store is about 2.7 miles southeast from the Britton Peak trailhead down Sawbill Trail. At Highway 61 turn right, and walk about a third of a mile down 61. The outfitter will be on your right.

Other nearby businesses and organizations: Coho Cafe, North Shore Commercial Fishing Museum, Bluefin Grill, Bluefin Bay on Lake Superior (hotel), Tofte General Store, Holiday gas station, Tofte Ranger Station for Superior National Forest, Zoar Lutheran Church, Waves of Lake Superior Spa, Grand Marais State Bank, Waters Edge Trading Company.

LUTSEN

Distance from the southern/northern terminuses: 215.6 mi/82.2 mi

Lutsen is about 4.5 miles down Ski Hill Road (Cook Co. Rd. 5) from the Lutsen Recreation Area trailhead. The resort has a shop with restaurants and limited gear options. The city of Lutsen has groceries, a post office, a laundromat and a hardware store.

I highly recommend hiking the spur trail to the Gondola because it runs terrifyingly close to the edge of the ridge, and crosses black-diamond ski runs. This spur offers a unique hiking experience for the SHT, amazing views and the Summit Chalet restaurant at its terminus.

POST OFFICE

Lutsen Post Office
5321 W. Highway 61
Lutsen, MN 55612
(218) 663-7323 • usps.com

Hours: Monday-Friday 8:30 a.m.-12:30 p.m. and 2:30-4:30 p.m., Saturday 8:45-9:45 a.m.

Holds resupply boxes for 10 days.

Distance from trail: About 3.8 miles from the Lutsen Recreation Area trailhead. Head southeast down Ski Hill Road and turn left on Highway 61. The post office will be on your left about 1.5 miles from the intersection. If you want to avoid walking on the highway, about half a mile before the intersection with 61 there is a snowmobile trail that runs about 1.5 miles and then connects with Steam Engine Road. Turn right on Steam Engine and follow it down toward 61. Conditions of this trail are unknown. Use at your own risk.

Other nearby organizations and businesses: Lockport Marketplace & Deli, Clearview General Store, Fika Coffee, laundromat, Isak Hansen Home and Hardware, Lutsen Lutheran Church, Lutsen Liquor Store, North Shore Federal Credit Union, Lutsen Resort, Caribou Highlands Resort, Papa Charlie's Saloon and Grill, The Mountain Shop at Lutsen Mountains.

RESUPPLY BOX

Lutsen Mountains Activity Center

450 Ski Hill Rd.
Lutsen, MN 55612
(218) 406-1320 • stay@lutsen.com

Hours: 10 a.m.-5 p.m. May 31-Oct. 20

Lutsen Mountains is able to accept resupply boxes at their Activity Center. No time limit, except for season dates listed above. Please use the following format to address the box:

Lutsen Mountains Activity Center
Attn: SHT Drop for Your Name <Estimated date of pick up>
450 Ski Hill Rd.
Lutsen, MN 55612

Distance from the trail: About .5 miles from the Lutsen Recreation Area trailhead. Head southeast down Ski Hill Road .5 miles. Eagle Ridge Resort will be on your right.

Other nearby organizations and businesses: The Mountain Shop at Lutsen Mountains, Lockport Marketplace & Deli, Post Office, Clearview General Store, Fika Coffee, laundromat, Isak Hansen Home and Hardware, Lutsen Lutheran Church, Lutsen Liquor Store, North Shore Federal Credit Union, Lutsen Resort, Caribou Highlands Resort, Papa Charlie's Saloon and Grill, Eagle Ridge Resort at Lutsen Mountains.

GROCERY

Clearview General Store

> 5323 Highway 61
> Lutsen, MN 55612
> (218) 663-7478 • clearviewgeneral.com

Hours: Winter season: 7 a.m.-8 p.m. Sunday-Thursday, and Fridays and Saturdays 7 a.m.-9 p.m. Summer season (Memorial Day through the end of October): 7 a.m.-9 p.m. Monday-Sunday.

The store is expanding its grocery options and will have more fresh foods. They also carry propane fuel, tents, sleeping pads, Superior Hiking Trail books, pet supplies, ice cream, and more. Clearview is also able to hold resupply boxes. Call ahead to arrange.

Distance from trail: About 3.8 miles from the Lutsen Recreation Area trailhead. Head southeast down Ski Hill Road and turn left on Highway 61. The store will be on your left in about 1.5 miles.

Other nearby organizations and businesses: Lockport Marketplace & Deli, Post Office, Fika Coffee, laundromat, Isak Hansen Home and Hardware, Lutsen Lutheran Church, Lutsen Liquor Store, North Shore Federal Credit Union, Lutsen Resort, Caribou Highlands Resort, Papa Charlie's Saloon and Grill, The Mountain Shop at Lutsen Mountains, Eagle Ridge Resort at Lutsen Mountains.

LAUNDRY

There is a laundromat in town, though it is not listed online and it doesn't appear to have a business sign or posted hours, but the laundromat is located two buildings west of TimberWolff Realty (5339 W. Highway 61, Lutsen, MN 55612).

Other nearby organizations and businesses: Lockport Marketplace & Deli, Post Office, Clearview General Store, Fika Coffee, Isak Hansen Home and Hardware, Lutsen Lutheran Church, Lutsen Liquor Store, North Shore Federal Credit Union, Lutsen Resort, Caribou Highlands Resort, Papa Charlie's Saloon and Grill, The Mountain Shop at Lutsen Mountains, Eagle Resort at Lutsen Mountains.

GEAR (LIMITED)

Isak Hansen Home and Hardware

> 4921 W. Highway 61
> Lutsen, MN 55612
> (218) 663-7201 • isakhansen.com

Hours: Monday-Friday 7:30 a.m.-5 p.m., Saturday 8 a.m.-4:30 p.m., and Sunday 9 a.m.-2 p.m.

They sell some camping gear: gas, HEET for alcohol stoves, tarps, batteries and flashlights.

Distance from the trail: About 5.6 miles from the Lutsen Recreation Area trailhead. Head southeast down Ski Hill Road and turn left on Highway 61. The store will be on your left in about 3.5 miles.

Other nearby organizations and businesses: Lockport Marketplace & Deli, Post Office, Clearview General Store, Fika Coffee, laundromat, Lutsen Lutheran Church, Lutsen Liquor Store, North Shore Federal Credit Union, Lutsen Resort, Caribou Highlands Resort, Papa Charlie's Saloon and Grill, The Mountain Shop at Lutsen Mountains, Eagle Ridge Resort at Lutsen Mountains.

The Mountain Shop

> 452 Ski Hill Rd.
> Lutsen, MN 55612
> (218) 663-7842 • themtnshopatlutsenmtns.com

Hours: Summer hours (Memorial Day until the 3rd weekend in October) are Monday-Sunday 10 a.m.-5 p.m. Winter hours are Monday-Friday 9 a.m.-4:30 p.m. and Saturday and Sunday 8:30 a.m.-4:30 p.m.

This shop is targeted more toward skiers, but there are gear options here like rain shells, warm layers and wool socks. They also stock some snacks like candy bars, granola and bars. Close by are Papa Charlie's Saloon & Grill and a deli.

Distance from the trail: About .5 miles from the Lutsen Recreation Area trailhead. Head southeast down Ski Hill Road .5 miles. The Mountain Shop will be on your left.

Other nearby organizations and businesses: Lockport Marketplace & Deli, Post Office, Clearview General Store, Fika Coffee, laundromat, Isak Hansen Home and Hardware, Lutsen Lutheran Church, Lutsen Liquor Store, North Shore Federal Credit Union, Lutsen Resort, Caribou Highlands Resort, Papa Charlie's Saloon and Grill, Eagle Ridge Resort at Lutsen Mountains.

OTHER
Fika Coffee

> 5327 W. Highway 61 (in the Clearview Building)
> Lutsen, MN 55612
> (218) 663-9055 • fikacoffee.com

Hours: Monday-Saturday 7 a.m.-5 p.m. and Sunday 7 a.m. to noon. Hours are seasonal. Check online before visiting.

Free wifi with purchase.

Distance from trail: About 3.8 miles from the Lutsen Recreation Area trailhead. Head southeast down Ski Hill Road and turn left on Highway 61. The store will be on your left in about 1.5 miles.

Other nearby organizations and businesses: Lockport Marketplace & Deli, Post Office, Clearview General Store, laundromat, Isak Hansen Home and Hardware, Lutsen Lutheran Church, Lutsen Liquor Store, North Shore Federal Credit Union, Lutsen Resort, Caribou Highlands Resort, Papa Charlie's Saloon and Grill, The Mountain Shop at Lutsen Mountains, Eagle Ridge Resort at Lutsen Mountains.

CASCADE LODGE

Distance from southern/northern terminuses: 230 mi/67.2 mi

About halfway between Lutsen and Grand Marais, Cascade Lodge offers another resupply option. They are willing to hold resupply boxes for hikers and are just .2 miles off the trail.

> 3719 W. Highway 61
> Lutsen, MN 55612
> (218) 387-1112 • cascadelodgemn.com

Hours: Monday-Sunday, 8 a.m.-8 p.m.

Price: $119-$419

The lodge offers everything from single rooms to cabins and vacation homes. They are willing to hold resupply boxes for thru-hikers who are not staying with them. One week past estimated arrival date, unclaimed boxes are moved to the lost and found, which is emptied each week. Please make sure your name is on the package, and your expected pickup date.

Distance from the trail: About .2 miles. Coming from the south, when you descend from Lookout Mountain, the SHT intersects with a ski trail that goes to Cascade Lodge. Turn right and follow the trail .2 miles to the lodge. There is a sign at the junction that points the way. Coming from the north, after you cross Cascade Creek, the SHT intersects with the ski trail that runs to the lodge. Turn left and follow the ski trail .2 miles. There is a sign at the junction that points the way.

Other nearby organizations and businesses: The lodge has a restaurant and pub onsite open the same hours as the lodge.

GRAND MARAIS

Distance from southern/northern terminuses: 246.3 mi/51.5 mi

Grand Marais wins "Best SHT Trail Town," in my opinion. There are too many amazing restaurants in Grand Marais to list. Have fun eating your way through town while you go about your chores. Grand Marais offers multiple grocery stores, a co-op, gear stores, laundromats, coffee galore, and an option to shower for $3 at the municipal campground. Grand Marais is the perfect town for a "nero," but Grand Marais is so fun, I highly recommend taking a zero, or even two.

POST OFFICE

Grand Marais Post Office
>117 E. Highway 61
>Grand Marais, MN 55604
>(218) 387-1020 • usps.com

Hours: Monday-Friday 9 a.m.-4 p.m., Saturday 9-11 a.m. and Sunday CLOSED

Able to hold resupply boxes for 30 days.

Distance from the trail: About 1.6 miles. From the trail, head southwest on the Gunflint Trail. Turn right on 5th Ave. Turn left on 4th St. and right onto 2nd Ave. E. The post office will be on your right.

Other nearby organizations and businesses: Gene's Foods, Subway, Grand Marais State Bank, Johnson's Foods.

GROCERY

Cook County Whole Foods Co-op

20 E. 1st St.
Grand Marais, MN 55604
(218) 387-2503 • cookcounty.coop
Hours: Monday-Sunday 9 a.m.-7 p.m. In July and August, the co-op is open Monday-Sunday 8 a.m.-8 p.m.

The co-op has a great bulk section with trail mix, dried soups, dried hummus mix, nuts, granola. You can buy what you need. They have a great selection of bars and other things hikers love. They also have a deli and a hot bar if you want to grab a meal while grabbing groceries.

Distance from the trail: About 1.7 miles. From the trail, head southwest on the Gunflint Trail. Turn right on 5th Ave. Turn left onto W. 2nd St. and right onto Broadway. Cross Highway 61 and turn left onto 1st St. The co-op will be on your right.

Other nearby organizations and businesses: Stone Harbor Wilderness Supply, Lake Superior Trading Post, World's Best Donuts, South of the Border Cafe, Buck's Hardware, Cook County Historical Museum, Sven and Ole's (pizza).

Gene's Foods

431 E. Highway 61
Grand Marais, MN 55604
(218) 387-1212 • genesfoods.com
Hours: Monday-Saturday 9 a.m.-7 p.m., Sunday CLOSED

Distance from trail: About 1.6 miles. From the trail, head southwest on the Gunflint Trail. Turn right onto 3rd Ave. E., left onto 6th St. and right on 4th Ave. E. Gene's will be on the left.

Other nearby organizations and businesses: Stone Harbor Wilderness Supply, Lake Superior Trading Post, World's Best Donuts, South of the Border Cafe, Buck's Hardware, Cook County Historical Museum.

Johnson's Foods

5 E. Highway 61
Grand Marais, MN 55604
(218) 387-2480 • johnsonsfoods.com
Hours: Monday-Saturday 7:30 a.m.-7 p.m., Sunday CLOSED

Distance from the trail: About 1.6 miles. From the trail, head southwest on the Gunflint Trail. Turn right onto 5th Ave. W., then left onto W. 2nd St. and right on Broadway. The store is at the intersection of Highway 61 and Broadway.

Other nearby organizations and businesses: Holiday, Hungry Hippie Tacos, South of the Border Cafe, Grand Marais Municipal Liquor Store, Grand Marais Public Library.

LAUNDRY

North Shore Laundromat

421 3rd Ave. W.
Grand Marais, MN 55604
(218) 387-1537
Hours: Open 24 hours, 7 days a week

Distance from trail: About 1.3 miles. From the trail, head southwest on the Gunflint Trail. Turn right on 5th Ave. The laundromat is at the intersection of 5th Ave. and 3rd St.

Other nearby organizations and businesses: Cook County North Shore Hospital & Care Center, Angry Trout, Sven and Ole's (pizza), Grand Marais Pharmacy.

Napa Laundromat

No address listed online, but it's right next to the North Shore Car Wash at 400 W. Highway 61.
Hours: Open 24 hours

Distance from trail: About 1.7 miles. From the trail, head southwest on the Gunflint Trail. Turn right on 3rd. Ave. E. and left onto Highway 61. The laundromat will be on the right.

Other nearby organizations and businesses: Post office, Subway, My Sister's Place, Gene's Foods.

GEAR

Stone Harbor Wilderness Supply

22 E. 1st St.
Grand Marais, MN 55604
(218) 387-3136 • stoneharborws.com
Hours: Monday-Saturday 9 a.m.-7 p.m. and Sunday 10 a.m.-6 p.m.

This store will have everything a thru-hiker needs: gear, fuel and more. They offer vegetarian and vegan backpacking food. Gear is usually priced at MSRP, which means it is similar to the prices you will find in major metro areas. Stone Harbor is also able to hold resupply boxes as long as needed, but ask hikers to pick up their box by a specified date, which can be negotiated with the store. Call to arrange. To ship resupply boxes, mail to P.O. Box 818, Grand Marais, MN 55604. Please include your name and expected arrival date on the box. In 2022, showers will be available for $5 or free with a minimum purchase of $20.

Distance from the trail: About 1.7 miles. From the trail, head southwest on the Gunflint Trail. Turn right onto 5th Ave. W., then left onto W. 2nd St. and right on Broadway. Cross Highway 61 and turn left onto 1st St. The store will be on the right.

Other nearby organizations and businesses: Cook County Whole Foods Co-op, Java Moose Espresso Cafe, Drury Lane Books, World's Best Donuts.

Lake Superior Trading Post

10 S. 1st. Ave. W.
Grand Marais, MN 55604
(218) 387-2020 • lakesuperiortradingpost.com

Hours: Summer hours (Memorial Day through Labor Day) are Monday-Saturday, 9 a.m.-8 p.m. and Sunday, 9 a.m.-5:30 p.m. Hours do change seasonally. Starting Labor Day, hours are Monday-Saturday 9 a.m.-6 p.m. and Sundays 9 a.m.-5 p.m. Off-season minimum hours are Monday-Thursday 10 a.m.-5 p.m. and Friday and Saturday, 9 a.m.-5:30 p.m., and Sundays 10 a.m.-5 p.m.

The trading post has everything a thru-hiker needs: gear, dehydrated meals, fuel and more. Maps for the SHT are available here, and they have a really good selection of hiking shoes, boots, socks, and base layers. The Trading Post is willing to hold resupply boxes at no charge. Please make sure your name and expected arrival date are on the box, and a phone number, if possible. The store only accepts boxes shipped via FedEx, UPS, and Spee-Dee. USPS boxes not accepted.

Distance from the trail: About 1.7 miles. From the trail, head southwest on the Gunflint Trail. Turn right right onto 5th Ave. W. , then left onto W. 2nd St. and left onto 1st Ave. W. The store will be on the left.

Other nearby organizations and businesses: Java Moose, Fireweed Bike Cooperative, World's Best Donuts, Joynes Ben Franklin.

SHOWER ONLY

Cook County YMCA

105 W. 5th St.
Grand Marais, MN 55604
(218) 387-3386
duluthymca.org/locations/cook-county-ymca

Hours: Monday-Friday 7 a.m.-7 p.m. and Saturday 9 a.m.-1 p.m.

The YMCA offers a day pass for $10 that allows the use of anything in the facility, including the showers and hot tub. If you're feeling sore, and need a soak, this would be a great option. Also, if you're not staying in town and just want a quick shower before heading back out on trail, this is a good option.

Distance from the trail: About 1.2 miles. From the trail, head southwest on the Gunflint Trail. Turn right on 5th Ave. W. and go one block to 5th St. E. Turn left and go four blocks to 1st Ave. W. The YMCA will be on your left.

Other nearby organizations and businesses: Cook County Community Center, Cook County North Shore Hospital, North Shore Laundromat.

LODGING

Grand Marais Campground and Marina

114 S. 8th Ave. W.
Grand Marais, MN 55604
(218) 387-1712 • grandmaraisrecreationarea.com

Hours: Between June 15 and Sept. 15, Monday-Sunday 8 a.m.-8 p.m. Outside of the summer season, the office opens every day at 8 a.m. but closes at different times. The campground has non-reservable walk-in sites for both backpackers and bike tourers. There are a couple weekends that require a two-night stay. Call for more information.

Price: $25-$32

Hikers not staying at the campground are able to shower for $3. Please pay in office first.

Distance from trail: About 1.7 miles. From the trail crossing at the Gunflint Trail, turn right and head southwest toward town. Turn right on 5th Ave. Turn right on Highway 61. Turn left onto W. 8th Ave.

Other nearby organizations and businesses: North House Folk School, Grand Marais Pharmacy, Dockside Fish Market.

Other things to know: The campground has free wifi in the office. You'll walk right past the North Shore Laundromat on your way to the campground if you want to stop and do laundry first. Some dates require a two-night stay. (Bike trail drop-in sites open to backpackers too?)

The Hungry Hippie Farm & Hostel

> 401 Co. Rd. 14
> Grand Marais, MN 55604
> (218) 387-2256 • hungryhippiehostel.com

Hours: Contact for more information

Price: $35-$159

The hostel has a campground, private rooms, and a suite that sleeps six. They no longer have a bunkhouse. The price includes access to the communal fire pit and the new shower house. The hostel accepts dogs, but requires hikers with dogs to stay in the campground or a single room (#5) and pay an extra $20 pet fee. The campground has plenty of great trees for hammocks. Hikers who aren't staying at the hostel are welcome to shower for $5 and can also do a load of laundry for $5. The Hungry Hippie is also willing to hold resupply boxes for three weeks. This would be a great resupply option if you're looking to completely avoid going into town.

Distance from the trail: At trail junction with Cook Co. Rd. 14, turn left (north) and go 1 mile. This turn off can be confusing because in the SHT guide, the eastern end of 14 intersects with the Lake Walk. Take the 14 that heads north from the trailhead near the Kimball Creek campsite.

Distance from southern/northern terminuses: 258.7 mi/ 39.1 mi

Other nearby organizations and businesses: None.

HOVLAND

Distance from southern/northern terminuses: 283.7 mi/15.1 mi* (*includes mileage for in-and-out hike of northern terminus)

Hovland is a small town. For thru-hikers, the only amenities at this location are a deli and post office. If you're planning to continue hiking onto the Border Route Trail, this would be your final place to resupply unless you arrange for a shuttle to meet you at the northern terminus of the SHT or hike straight from Grand Marais to a resupply drop at an outfitter along the BRT.

POST OFFICE

Hovland Post Office

12 Arrowhead Trail
Hovland, MN 55606
(218) 475-2286 • usps.com

Hours: Monday-Friday 11 a.m.-3 p.m., and Saturday 9 a.m. to noon, and Sunday CLOSED.

Able to hold general delivery boxes for 30 days.

Distance from the trail: About 3.2 miles. At the Arrowhead Trail parking lot, turn south and walk 3.2 miles to the post office. The post office will be on your left.

Other nearby organizations and businesses: Chicago Bay Marketplace-Bakery, Trinity Lutheran Church.

GROCERY (LIMITED)

Chicago Bay Marketplace-Bakery

4971 Highway 61
Hovland, MN 55606
(218) 475-2253

Hours: Memorial Day through Labor Day,
Tuesday-Saturday 8:30 a.m.-5 p.m. and Sunday CLOSED.
Hours vary during the off-season.

Distance from the trail: About 3.5 miles. At the Arrowhead Trail parking lot, turn south and walk about 3.2 miles to Highway 61.
Turn right onto 61 and walk another third of a mile. The deli will be on your right.

Other nearby organizations and businesses: Post office, Trinity Lutheran Church.

Other things to know: Limited groceries available, coffee, beer, and a variety of amazing fresh baked pastries, bread, pizza and more.

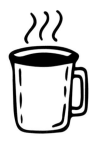

The end, a beginning?

When I reached the northern terminus, I was so damn proud of myself, and so damn sad. My great adventure on the SHT was over. I sat on the 270 Degree Overlook for an hour, and watched the woods below. Not having any more trail to hike felt surreal. I replayed my memories, trying to cement it all in my mind.

The vast majority of my mornings on trail, I was profoundly grateful to be alive, and invigorated by the beauty around me. There were a few days when I badly missed my family and friends, and loneliness deadened my joy. In response, I would take a mindful moment, breathe deeply of the fresh woodland air, listen to the birds singing and the wind sighing in the trees. I would note the golden quality of light, and how eager my body felt to hike another day. My gratitude to be thru-hiking would last until sheer exhaustion set in at the end of the day.

I learned a lot of practical things on trail — how to manage being plagued by bugs, keep my body happy, and throw a bear rope with precision. I learned that I love to hike in the rain when I'd dreaded the idea, that the night noises of the woods become as familiar as the creaking of an old house. I revelled in the capability of my body to wander great distances. I also gained a powerful connection with nature that I suspect will shape the rest of my life.

I hope this guide will help to grant you similar lessons, and see you through to the very end of the trail. I hope it will galvanize people who've pushed down a desire to thru-hike because the logistics feel overwhelming or complicated. I also hope this guide will inspire in you a great love of long-distance hiking, a desire to protect and support this trail, and wild spaces. I wish you all happy, challenging, life-changing hiking.

Annie Nelson